EPA 300 R 01 002
February 2001
http://es.epa.gov/oeca/main/ej/nejacpub.html

ENVIRONMENTAL JUSTICE AND COMMUNITY-BASED HEALTH MODEL DISCUSSION AND RECOMMENDATIONS REPORT

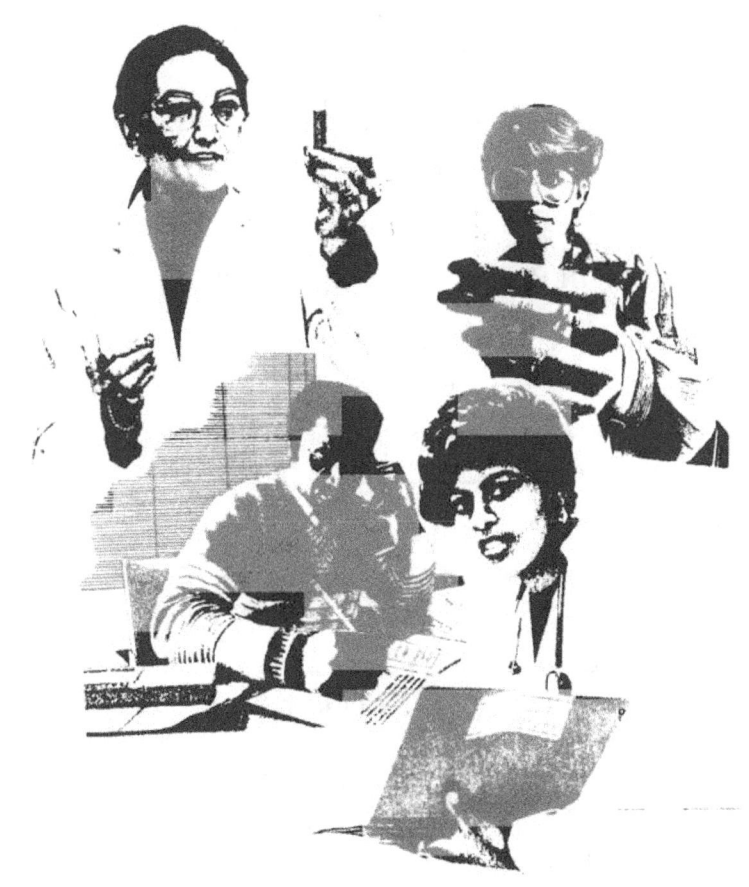

Prepared by the

National Environmental Justice Advisory Council

A Federal Advisory Committee to the U.S. Environmental Protection Agency

Tips for the Reader

The references referred to in this report are coded as follows:
Roman numerals "I-IV" refer to the transcripts of the NEJAC sessions conducted on December 23-26, 2000. The transcript from December 24th (II) is a in appendix III.E. Each report page contains four transcript pages.

Roman numeral "V" refers to "A Synopsis of Stakeholder Representatives' Views Regarding Community-Based Health Research Models Report, May 15, 2000 and is in appendix III.C.

Roman numeral "VI" refers to the "Indigenous Peoples Subcommittee, *Recommendations Concerning the Environmental Health and Research Needs Within Indian Country and Alaska Native Villages*, August 14, 2000 and is in appendix III.D.

Roman numeral "VII" refers to the written recommendations submitted by the Southwest Network for Environmental and Economic Justice, during public comment, May 23, 2000 and is in appendix III.E.

"HRS" refers to the synopsis of the May 25, 2000 NEJAC Health and Research Subcommittee meeting and is in appendix III.B.

The number following the roman numeral refers to the specific page of the document referenced.

Documents "I-VI" and "HRS" can also be found at EPA's website at:
http://www.epa.gov/oeca/main/ej/nejacpub.html

"VII" is not available in electronic format.

Disclaimer

This report and recommendations have been written as a part of the activities of the National Environmental Justice Advisory Council, a public advisory committee providing external policy information and advice to the Administrator and other officials of the United States Environmental Protection Agency (EPA). The Council is structured to provide balanced, expert assessment of issues related to environmental justice.

This report has not been reviewed for approval by the EPA and, hence, its contents and recommendations do not necessarily represent the views and polices of the EPA, nor of other agencies in the Executive Branch of the federal government, nor does mention of trade names or commercial products constitute a recommendation for use.

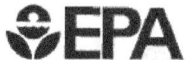 **NATIONAL ENVIRONMENTAL JUSTICE ADVISORY COUNCIL**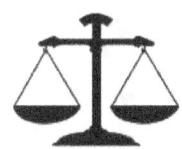

February 8, 2001

Administrator Christine Todd Whitman
U.S. Environmental Protection Agency
1200 Pennsylvania Avenue, NW
Washington, DC 20004

Dear Administrator Whitman,

Please find attached a copy of the report entitled *"Environmental Justice and Community-Based Health Model Discussion: A Report on the Public Meeting Convened by the National Environmental Justice Advisory Council, May 23 - 26, 2000."*

EPA, through its Office of Environmental Justice, asked the National Environmental Justice Advisory Council (NEJAC) to provide advice and recommendations on the following questions:

(1) What strategies and areas of research[1] should be pursued to achieve more effective, integrated community-based health assessment, intervention, and prevention efforts?

(2) How should these strategies be developed, implemented and evaluated so as to ensure substantial participation, integration and collaboration among federal agencies, in partnership with: impacted communities; public health, medical and environmental professionals; academic institutions; state, tribal and local governments; and the private sector?

(3) How can consideration of socioeconomic status and cultural factors: (a) contribute to health disparities and cumulative and disproportionate environmental effects; and (b) be incorporated into community health assessments?

In short, this report reflects the advice and recommendations that resulted from pre-meeting preparation (i.e., interviews) and on-site discussions and public comments. The breath of the discussions were exemplified by individuals and/or organizations that either provided comments, suggestions or recommendations on what EPA could and/or should consider in addressing these health-related issues. As a whole, it sets forth a number of policy recommendations for consideration by EPA and other federal, state and local agencies to consider.

These recommendations are listed under five (5) key recommendations that were identified to be the dominant themes surfaced repeatedly among the stakeholders in both interviews and public

---

[1] Research in this context encompasses a broad range of studies that may include basic science, applied research, and data collection. These may be carried out by: federal, state, tribal or local governments; universities; communities; industry; and/or individuals.

testimony. It is recognized that to accomplish these goals, EPA will need to take the lead and/or work in companion with other federal agencies in a collaborative manner. Consequently, NEJAC recommends that the *Administrator*:

- <u>Promote Better Understanding of "Community-Based Participatory Research Models"</u> - - EPA and other federal agencies need to better understand the approach and usefulness of "community-based participatory research models" and the importance of including prevention and intervention components in these projects.

- <u>Place Greater Emphasis on Translating Current and Future Scientific Knowledge Into Positive Action</u> - - EPA and other federal agencies may fail to act on a problem because of an inability to "prove" a casual relationship. Having said that, greater emphasis needs to be placed on translating current and future scientific knowledge into more positive action at the policy and community level (i.e., what can the government do to help, even though the exact science is not readily available or known).

- <u>Promote More Effective Interagency Collaboration and Cooperation</u> - - EPA and other federal agencies should establish more extensive formal and informal interagency mechanisms to help assure that the necessary expertise and other resources are brought to bear on eliminating health disparities and disproportionate exposures. Part of this process would better define responsibilities and available resources for dealing with specific problems and issues.

- <u>Include Socioeconomic and Cultural Factors in Health Assessments</u> - - EPA and other federal agencies need to examine the impact and significance of socioeconomic and cultural factors on health disparities. Then, as appropriate, include these factors in health assessment, intervention, and prevention strategies.

- <u>Respond to Urgent Needs of Medically Underserved Communities</u> - - EPA and other federal agencies need to further examine the most significant needs of medically underserved communities. The mechanisms established to address these concerns should be brought to bear to eliminate or reduce disparities in health care access and improving environmental health education.

The process for developing this report included the formation of a multi-stakeholder recommendations Working Group that attempted to capture and compile the presentations and discussions that occurred during the NEJAC meeting. Also, attached is a list of the names and affiliations of all those who served on this Working Group.

We are pleased to present this report to you for your review, consideration, response and action.

Sincerely,

Peggy Shepard
Acting, Chair, NEJAC

NEJAC MAY 2000 MEETING REPORT
ENVIRONMENTAL JUSTICE AND COMMUNITY-BASED HEALTH
MODEL DISCUSSION

Table of Contents

I. **BACKGROUND** 1
   I.A   Meeting Issues 3
   I.B   Broad Recommendations 6
II. **RECOMMENDATIONS** 7
   II.A   Promote better understanding of the approach and usefulness of "community-based participatory research models" and the importance of including prevention and intervention components in these models 7
      II.A.1   Background 7
         II.A.1.a   Participation 8
         II.A.1.b   Using community knowledge 9
         II.A.1.c   Building capability 10
         II.A.1.d   Intervention/Prevention 11
         II.A.1.e   Barriers 11
         II.A.1.f   Lack of agreed upon definitions 13
      II.A.2   Recommendations (Promote better understanding of the approach and usefulness of "community-based participatory research models"...) 13
   II.B   Translating Current and Future Scientific Knowledge Into Positive Action 16
      II.B.1   Background 16
      II.B.2   Recommendations (Translating Current and Future Scientific Knowledge Into Positive Action) 17
   II.C   More Effective Interagency Collaboration and Cooperation 21
      II.C.1   Background 21
      II.C.2   Recommendations (More Effective Interagency Collaboration and Cooperation) 22
   II.D   Including Socioeconomic and Cultural Factors in Health Assessments 24
      II.D.1   Background 24
      II.D.2   Recommendations (Including Socioeconomic and Cultural Factors in Health Assessments) 27
   II.E   Responding to the Urgent Needs of Medically Underserved Communities 28
      II.E.1   Background 28
      II.E.2   Recommendations (Responding to the Urgent Needs of Medically Underserved Communities) 28

III. Appendices 33

  III.A Recommendations Work Group 33

  III.B May 2000 NEJAC HEALTH AND RESEARCH SUBCOMMITTEE Meeting
         Synopsis (HRS) 35

  III.C A Synopsis of Stakeholder Representatives' Views Regarding Community-Based
         Health Research Models Report, May 15, 2000 (V) 39

  III.D Indigenous Peoples Subcommittee, *Recommendations Concerning the
         Environmental Health and Research Needs Within Indian Country and Alaska Native
         Villages,* August 14, 2000 (VI) 69

  III.E Written Recommendations submitted by the Southwest Network for Environmental
         and Economic Justice, May 23, 2000 (VII) 83

  III.F Transcript - May 25, 2000 NEJAC Meeting (II) 85

NEJAC MAY MEETING REPORT INTRODUCTION

I. BACKGROUND

According to the 1997 Strategic Plan, the mission of the U.S. Environmental Protection Agency (EPA) is to protect human health and to safeguard the natural environment–air, water, and land–upon which all life depends. Although the EPA has made significant progress in achieving healthier, sustainable environments, the Strategic Plan states that "environmental programs during the past two decades may not always have benefitted all communities or all populations equally. Many minority, low-income, and Native American communities have raised concerns that they suffer a disproportionate burden of health due to the siting of multiple pollution sources in their communities. Environmental programs do not adequately address these disproportionate exposures to pesticides, lead or other toxic chemicals at home and on the job." Specifically, the Strategic Plan emphasizes the following:

- Approximately 126 million people live in areas of non-attainment for pollutants which have health-based standards.

- Contaminated water poses a special risk to children, the elderly[1], women of childbearing age and sub-populations who fish for food or sport.

- Almost 1 million children under the age of six still have elevated blood lead levels.

- 20 to 30 million Americans have asthma, leading to the death of approximately 4,000 people per year. There are high incidences of asthma among children, especially those from low-income and minority communities.

- 10 million children annually may become ill from contaminated air in schools[1].

Protecting the health of all communities presents a formidable challenge for the EPA. However, this responsibility does not rest solely with the EPA, but is shared with other Federal departments and agencies as well as state and local governments.

In January 2000, the U.S. Surgeon General issued the publication, "Healthy People 2010–Understanding and Improving Health." One of the goals of Healthy People 2010 is to eliminate health disparities among different segments of the population, including differences that occur by race or ethnicity, education or income. Some examples of these health disparities include:

- The infant mortality rate among African-Americans is still more than double that of whites.

- Heart disease death rates are more than 40 percent higher for African-Americans than for

---

[1] EPA's 2000 Strategic Plan

whites.

- The death rate for all cancers is 30 percent higher for African-Americans than for whites. For prostate cancer, it is more than double that for whites.

- African-American women have a higher death rate from breast cancer despite having a mammography screening rate that is higher than that for white women.

- The Hispanic cancer experience also differs from that of the non-Hispanic white population, with Hispanics having higher rates of cervical, esophageal, gallbladder, and stomach cancers. New cases of female breast and lung cancers are increasing among Hispanics, who are diagnosed at later stages and have lower survival rates than whites.

- In New York City, African American, Hispanic, and low-income populations have been found to have hospitalization and death rates from asthma 3 to 5 times higher than those for all New York City residents.

- Death from asthma is two to six times more likely to occur among African Americans and Hispanics than among whites.

- Although childhood lead poisoning occurred in all population groups, the risk was higher for persons having low income, living in older housing, and belonging to certain racial and ethic groups. For example, among non-Hispanic black children living in homes built before 1946, 22 percent had elevated blood lead levels.

- Hispanics have higher rates of high blood pressure than non-Hispanic whites.

- American Indians and Alaska Natives have an infant death rate almost double that for whites.

- The rate of diabetes for American Indians and Alaska Natives is more than twice that for whites.

- In 1996, a disproportionate number of Hispanics and Asian and Pacific Islanders lived in areas that failed to meet these standards compared with whites, African Americans, and American Indians or Alaska Natives.

The Healthy People 2010 report identifies environmental quality as a leading health indicator. It reveals that an estimated 25 percent of preventable illnesses worldwide can be attributed to poor environmental quality. In the U.S., air pollution is estimated to be associated with 50,000 premature deaths and $40 to $50 billion in health related costs annually.

Other entities recognized that such disturbing statistics needed to be addressed by government public health agencies in a more coordinated and focused approach. For example, in 1999, the Institute of Medicine issued its report, *Toward Environmental Justice: Research, Education and Health Policy Needs*. The report's four major recommendations called for the following:

(1) A coordinated effort among federal, state, and local public health agencies is needed to improve the collection and coordination of environmental health information and to better link it to specific populations and communities of concern;

(2) Public health research related to environmental justice should engender three principles: improve the science base, involve the affected populations, and communicate the results to all stakeholders;

(3) Environmental justice, in general, and specific environmental hazards, in particular, should be the focus of educational efforts to improve the understanding of these issues between community residents and health professionals, including medical, nursing, and public health practitioners; and

(4) In instances in which the science is incomplete with respect to environmental health and justice issues, policymakers are urged to exercise caution on behalf of the affected communities, particularly those that have the least access to medical, political, and economic resources, taking reasonable precautions to safeguard against or minimize adverse health outcomes.

Federal agencies have also heard, poignant testimony from the residents of adversely affected communities, who suffer the illnesses enumerated above. These health concerns have been expressed by the public in numerous meetings, conferences and forums conducted on the subject of environmental justice during the past decade. One such meeting was the 1994 "Interagency Symposium on Health Research and Needs to Ensure Environmental Justice" (Crystal City, Virginia, February 10-12, 1994), which brought together for the first time significant numbers of community residents and representatives from Federal agencies to dialogue around public health issues related to environmental justice.

In light of the above, the Office of Environmental Justice asked the National Environmental Justice Advisory Council (NEJAC) to hold a meeting focusing on strategies to ensure disease prevention and health improvement in communities, particularly minority and low-income communities. To that end, the NEJAC convened an issue-oriented, focused public meeting in Atlanta, Georgia (May 23-26, 2000).

The NEJAC is the EPA's formal advisory committee on matters of environmental justice. Its charter provides that the NEJAC is to provide independent advice to the Administrator on areas which may include the direction, criteria, scope and adequacy of the Agency's scientific research and demonstration projects relating to environmental justice.

I.A   Meeting Issues

The meeting focused on Federal efforts to secure disease prevention and health improvement in communities where health disparities may result from, or be exacerbated by, disproportionate effects of environmental pollutants. The following questions were considered:

(1) What strategies and areas of research should be pursued to achieve more effective, integrated community-based health assessment, intervention, and prevention efforts?

(2) How should these strategies be developed, implemented and evaluated so as to ensure substantial participation, integration and collaboration among Federal agencies, in partnership with: impacted communities; public health, medical and environmental professionals; academic institutions; state, tribal and local governments; and the private sector?

(3) How can consideration of socioeconomic vulnerabilities: (a) contribute to better understanding of health disparities and cumulative and disproportionate environmental effects; and (b) be incorporated into community health assessments?

Prior to the May NEJAC meeting, 21 stakeholders who represented academia (8); industry/business (1); Federal agencies (6), state health and environmental agencies (3); and community groups and tribal entities (3) were interviewed. These stakeholders had all participated in community-based activity, including funding research projects, conducting assessment, intervention, evaluation, and/or prevention activities with communities, or by working directly in and with communities. The pre-meeting report, which summarizes the interviews is Appendix III.C, "A Synopsis of Stakeholder Representatives' Views Regarding Community-Based Health Research Models Report," and was disseminated at the May 2000 NEJAC meeting.

A number of general themes resulted from the stakeholder interviews as well as the meeting and are briefly discussed below:

In general, stakeholders agreed that there is a need to:

(1) develop an integrated model to address community-based health needs and that participation, assessment, intervention/prevention should be the critical components of a community-based health research model. (II - 234[2]; II - 275-6; V - 6; V - 10);

---

[2]**Note: The following reports were used as references (document and page number) for this report**:
I - Transcript - Tuesday, May 23, 2000, NEJAC meeting
II - Transcript - Wednesday, May 24, 2000, NEJAC meeting
III - Transcript - Health and Research and Waste and Facility Siting Joint Subcommittee
    Meeting, Thursday, May 25, 2000
IV - Transcript - Friday, May 26, 2000, NEJAC meeting
V - A Synopsis of Stakeholder Representatives' Views Regarding Community-Based Health Research Models Report, May 15, 2000

(2) create partnerships among stakeholders groups and that activities conducted in the community must involve the community as an equal partner. (V - 5; V - 7; II - 274; II - 58; II - 229);

(3) have Federal agencies learn to become partners with each other, as this would be more conducive to successful partnering with communities and other stakeholders. (II - 47; II - 53; II - 72; II - 109; II - 229; II - 267; II - 261; V - 14);

(4) whenever possible and appropriate, include state, local, and tribal governments in collaborative efforts to address human health and environmental justice issues, particularly with respect to data collection and monitoring. (VI-6, 7, 9)

(5) implement intervention and prevention programs, where the need exists, even though a direct causal relationship between exposure and health effects is not currently proven. (II - 182; II - 140); and

(6) consider socioeconomic, cultural, and traditional practices as factors when assessing and addressing community health concerns, since there is ample evidence of the association between these factors and health effects. (V - 12; II - 104; II - 187-8; I - 194; II - 197; II - 257; II - 194).

The stakeholders also identified barriers to both determination of causal relationships and to successful community-based health research models. Barriers to the determination of causal relationships included:

(1) the absence of human exposure and health surveillance information;

(2) the lack of health data to better elucidate socioeconomic and racial factors;

(3) that analyzing health impacts "one chemical at a time" precludes an understanding of cumulative environmental and human health effects;

(4) lack of awareness of community cultural values;

VI - Indigenous Peoples Subcommittee, *Recommendations Concerning the Environmental Health and Research Needs Within Indian Country and Alaska Native Villages*, August 14, 2000
VII - Written recommendations submitted by the Southwest Network for Environmental and Economic Justice, May 23, 2000
HRS - HEALTH AND RESEARCH SUBCOMMITTEE Meeting Synopsis, May 25, 2000
Some references are repeated in more than one section, because of applicability in both places; these are indicated by •• when repeated.

(5)   not knowing how to peer review participatory research;

(6)   need to establish funding mechanisms for community-based participatory health research; and

(7)   communication problems. (I - 37-8; I - 57; II - 55-6; II - 117-8; II - 280; II - 133-4; II - 291-2; II - 241; II - 251-3; IV - 188)

The recommendations appearing in this report reflect the advice and recommendations that resulted from: 1) the pre-meeting interviews; 2) panels, public comments, and discussion occurring during the May NEJAC meeting; 3) almost three months of conference calls and correspondence among the thirteen members of the "Recommendations Work Group" (listed in appendix III.A) working with EPA and some other Federal agency staff; and 4) a review round of a draft and conference call, followed by a ballot round by the NEJAC Council.

On November 22, 2000, President Clinton signed legislation that should help the Government follow many recommendations contained in this report. The Health Care Fairness Act is meant to improve the ability to deal with disparities in health based on race and ethnicity. The Act allocates more than $150 million to a new National Center for Research on Minority Health and Health Disparities within the National Institutes of Health. The legislation gives the Center four primary functions:

1)   The Director of the Center will participate with other Institute and Center Directors to determine policy and initiatives at NIH dealing with health disparity research;

2)   The Center will act as a catalyst for strategic planning for the entire NIH and the Director will be the primary federal official with responsibility for monitoring all minority health research conducted or supported by NIH;

3)   The Director of the Center has the authority to make peer-reviewed grants in areas of promising research, which are not addressed by the existing centers and institutes at NIH; and

4)   Establish a new program to support research excellence at those academic health centers which have demonstrated a historic commitment to studying and addressing diseases which disproportionately affect Americans in racial and ethnic minorities.

The legislation also allocates resources in increasing medical training for minorities.

I.B   Broad Recommendations

Based upon the meeting, the NEJAC has developed 5 broad recommendations (below) as well as a number of more detailed sub-recommendations that will be forwarded to the Administrator:

(1) EPA and other Federal agencies need to promote better understanding of the approach and usefulness of "community-based participatory research models" and the importance of including prevention and intervention components in these models;

(2) EPA and other Federal agencies may fail to act on a problem because of an inability to "prove" a casual relationship to health disparities. Greater emphasis needs to be placed on translating current scientific knowledge into positive action at the policy and community level (i.e., what can the government do to help, even though we don't have absolute proof);

(3) EPA and other Federal agencies should establish more extensive formal and informal interagency mechanisms to help assure that the necessary expertise and other resources are brought to bear on eliminating health disparities and disproportionate exposures. This process should better define responsibilities and available resources for dealing with specific problems and issues;

(4) EPA and other Federal agencies need to examine the impact and significance of socioeconomic factors, cultural and traditional values and practices on health disparities. Then, as appropriate, include these factors in developing health assessment, intervention, and prevention strategies; and

(5) EPA and other Federal agencies need to further examine the most significant needs of medically underserved communities. The mechanisms established in (3) above should then be used to eliminate or reduce disparities in access to health care and improving environmental health education.

II. RECOMMENDATIONS

Five (5) key recommendations surfaced repeatedly in the pre-meeting interviews and the panel discussions, public comments and the Health and Research Subcommittee meeting at the May NEJAC Meeting. This section contains background information on each of the recommendations and identifies related sub-recommendations.

II.A Promote better understanding of the approach and usefulness of "community-based participatory research models" and the importance of including prevention and intervention components in these models

II.A.1 Background

A longstanding area of discussion (and disagreement) has been the concept of "community-based health research." A major goal of this meeting was to get input as to how to best define and implement community-based health research.

The resulting dialogue has been divided into six parts for purposes of developing recommendations: (1) participation; (2) using community knowledge; (3) building capability; (4) intervention; (5) barriers; and (6) lack of agreed upon definitions.

II.A.1.a **Participation** - A major issue has been whether or not community participation was necessary to conduct successful community-based research and at what level that participation should occur.

- *There was almost unanimous agreement on the part of stakeholders that the community, or a community-based organization was the most critical component for a successful partnership. (V - 5)*

- *"...I don't think any of those (research projects) targeted to under-served communities can be done without partnership with that community. I think we have lots of evidence over the last 20 or 30 years that community-based research interventions don't work as well as community-based participatory research interventions...and so I think that partnership is essential..." (Jon Kerner, II - 274)*

- *"doing work in Harlem without ever having formed a partnership yet with anybody in the community. That wasn't the way to do it, and I learned that pretty rapidly..." (Patrick Kinney, II - 58)*

- *"....we need to keep improving the way we deal with communities and the way we generally develop our partnerships..." (Henry Falk, II - 229)*

Within the issue of participation, three sub-issues emerged:
(1) Should industry be a partner in community-based participatory health research?

- *A few representatives......felt that industry/business should be included in the partnership, in order to achieve success......one stakeholder from academia was very vocal **against** bringing industry to the partnership.....In contrast, a stakeholder from the state health/environmental agency stated that "...industry plays a key role as a stakeholder in this process...industry is not explicitly included in the process...they should not be considered a barrier, but they should be included in the partnership...." (V - 5)*

(2) There is a need to establish accountability and trust among the partners.

- *"...partnerships will work if accountability and structure are incorporated into the process...." (V - 5)*

- *According to one Federal stakeholder, "...trust is a critical element in any partnership...if you outline what you are going to do, do what you say will do and say what you cannot do, that will go a long way toward establishing trust and credibility...." (V - 5)*

(3) There's a concern about the lag time in communication of research or assessment results to the community.

- *"... we have a lag time between the translation of the science and its use in community education and prevention. A big issue for us. I would also hope that the Health and Research Subcommittee would kind of take a look at that issue and give us some of their concerns and some suggestions." (Michael Sage, II - 252)*

    II.A.1.b   Using community knowledge - One of the most significant arguments for partnering with the community is using the knowledge and abilities of the community.

- *"....some of the best ideas for doing research really arise from the community because they are in a much better position than the researchers are to understand what the real issues are." (Patrick Kinney, II - 59)*

- *.....partnering with communities to document environmental hazards and better data collection from communities will help to identify areas of need and help to improve methods on providing healthcare. (Rueben Warren, HRS)*

- *"...Providing a mechanism for meaningful community involvement from the initial stages of the risk assessment throughout the entire study, developing an understanding of the background health status of the community, including various sub-populations, along with more thorough exposure pathway information and multiple exposure sources, we feel, can improve this so-called risk assessment process, and such information can be gathered through the community. The bottom line is that we the people who are on the front line being affected every day must be included in the processes of assessment, intervention, and certainly prevention..." (Mildred McClain, II - 346)*

- *"...But, again, we have some data gaps. ...We did a physical inventory -- physical inventory with our community members walking the streets to document and list everything that was in this quarter mile radius....." (Carlos Porras, II - 99-100)*

- *"...the community has to be at the table -- and particularly the impacted, the most impacted community -- has to be at the table because they are the experts. They may not have PhDs, but they are experts in what needs to happen as it relates to resolving and remediating and preventing and addressing these problems..." (Robert Bullard, II - 49)*

- *Make regulatory decisions and develop Federal policies affecting the health of AI/AN communities in consultation with Federally recognized tribes. To the extent possible, such decisions should be based not only on science, but also should address and incorporate the traditional knowledge of the AI/AN community. For example, limitations on the consumption of traditional foods due to pollution danger may trigger unique social, economic, and health problems within AI/AN communities. (VI - 9)*

II.A.1.c Building capability

A lot of discussion occurred around building capability in the communities; the capability to participate in the health assessment as well as any intervention efforts.

- *The foundation for this model would be developed with education, training or outreach to the community, to ensure that everyone is "...on the same page...." (V - 6)*

- *Henry Falk, Assistant Administrator, ATSDR, stated that whatever efforts take place, they need to be sustainable. Types of partnerships that need to be created might need to be broader to include education, etc. (HRS)*

- *".....from the community's perspective there's some obvious advantages.....in terms of getting good science and data that they can use for policy advocacy. It also can bring funding in that it can help train young people and also provide education to the wider community. (Patrick Kinney, II - 60)*

- *Promote the Federal policy of tribal self-determination and self-sufficiency by building environmental protection and environmental health capabilities of Federally recognized tribes so that they can participate fully and effectively in the protection of the human health and environmental of AI/AN communities. (VI - 4)*

Part of building community capability is the process of creating and sustaining trust and understanding among the partners.

- *The overwhelming majority of the stakeholders agreed that establishing trust and credibility is time and resource intensive, and that this should be recognized and acknowledged by all stakeholders. (V - 5)*

- *"...There are three key aspects of successful work between researchers and a community, and they are respect, equity, and empowerment. (Pat Wood, II - 118)*

Also discussed was the need to provide the time and resources to establish partnerships.

- *"......Again, I'd like to emphasize the importance of pilot funding. Small scale funding to form partnerships to generate initial data can be extremely effective, and we've had a lot of success with small-scale studies....These partnerships take time to develop and they gradually develop over time.* (Patrick Kinney, II - 63)

Mentioned frequently was the need to sustain the community capability.

- *"There also has to be ongoing funding, dependable long-term funding."* (Patrick Kinney, II - 63)
- *"....whatever efforts take place they need to be sustainable."* (Henry Falk, HRS)

II.A.1.d Intervention/Prevention - A number of stakeholders stressed the need for the community to be significantly involved in all intervention/prevention efforts.

- *"...The community-based prevention and intervention research projects are designed to expand our knowledge and understanding of the potential causes and solutions for environmental related disorders and enhance the capability of the communities to participate in the development of research approaches and intervention strategies.* (Charles Wells, II-234)

- *"...I don't think you can implement an intervention without community-based efforts. If you're really going to implement...interventions, ultimately they come down to community-based efforts, truly."* (Michael Sage, II-275-6)

II.A.1.e Barriers - There was a lot of discussion relating to the barriers that currently inhibit the productivity of community-based participatory research projects. The most frequently mentioned barrier was the lack of awareness/consideration of cultural issues:

- *"...We also have a real lack of understanding of a lot of the cultural issues. When we actually end up getting involved directly in community-based efforts, we have lots bridges to gap in understanding cultural issues when we do go out into the field because oftentimes we do our work in Atlanta and miss the perception of the cultural issues in the community."* (Michael Sage, II-253)

- *"... if you want to work with our community, you must understand our culture, you must understand our religion, you must respect that -- and I'll go on to that in a little bit. These principles were things that we, as the academics, were taught by the community."* (David Carpenter, II - 117)

- *"I think ATSDR needs is to be a little more understanding of the culture of the community that they're going into. One of the health studies or assessments that they did in the*

community is they came, they started knocking on doors, and told the people they were interviewing, we'll give you $10 for your interview. The community started calling me and they were very upset because they felt that, you know, here they had family that was sick and dying, they had people that were -- that the families had died and they felt, well, what are they offering me $10 for? Is this what my family is worth to them, $10? So, you know, that is -- that was a slap in the face to offer them that. You know, $10 or any kind of money. They would have done it for free......So here's another cultural thing. In the Mexican community -- and this is the old people that I have seen and I have heard -- is when a person is dying, "oh, did you hear so and so has been suffering so much, she's got cancer. I wonder what sin she committed that she is suffering so much and God is punishing her."
(Rose Augustine, II - 280)

- *"....if you want to work with our community, you must understand our culture, you must understand our religion, you must respect that...."* (David Carpenter, II - 117)

- *".....its respect for culture, for tradition. It's respect for religion."* (David Carpenter, II - 118)

A barrier raised by a number of stakeholders was how to peer review technical products of the community-based participatory health research:

- *"....how do peer reviewers see community participation in research, truly...and from a community's perspective what are the things that community -- and I think this panel addressed some of it -- but what kind of community review is necessary on researchers and what are the criteria, so to speak, that each bring to the table in looking at each other. I ask this because I know that there are fundamental problems in the scientific community with true community input and there are fundamental problems in the community with the role that academics have played historically there.* (Michael Gelobter, II-133-4)

- *"...Who are your peers? I mean, if they're community-based partners, you need community-based folks doing the review. And we know that. But then getting a common understanding between reviewers about what's good science and what's good community-based research is also a challenge."* (Jon Kerner, II-291-2)

- *"It's very difficult science to get through peer review, and this is one of the challenges we face in the research community."* (Jon Kerner, II-241)

A third significant barrier mentioned involves how agencies are funded and how those funding mechanisms limit the ability to target monies for community-based participatory health research.

- *"...Some of the barriers I see in working with us is (that) our funding is very disease-*

> *specific and very issue-specific, meaning our funding comes from Congress targeted to asthma. That boxes then into just dealing with asthma. Funding comes for lead; it then boxes it into dealing with lead. I see that as a barrier in working with communities because it doesn't give us much leeway in working other issues that are often of more concern to communities...." " We have a lack of direct community access.....Most of our programs are run through state health departments and local health departments and we have very few efforts that are really actually direct community-based efforts......aligning our scientific expertise with community-based efforts has been a barrier for us."* (Michael Sage, II - 251-2)

- *They further stated that "...until the funding process changes, the research needed to do work in communities needs to go through academic institutions...."* (V - 5)

Another barrier is *the lack of a thorough understanding among Federal agency staff and managers of Federal Indian law and policies, tribal culture, and the unique governmental structure of Federally recognized Indian tribes, including Alaska Native villages.* (VI-10)

II.A.1.f Lack of agreed upon definitions

The lack of agreement upon definitions was an issue that was a constant part of this meeting, since its initial conception. These definitions include "community-based participatory health research" as well as each of the individual words (i.e., community; community-based; participatory; and research).

- *A number of stakeholders discussed the definition of 'community'. Some non-community stakeholders pointed out that there should be a mechanism to define community.....a stakeholder from the Federal Government stated that, "...leadership in communities must be defined by communities...we should not try to define community leadership, let them (the community) identify leaders...."*
(V - 5)

II.A.2 Recommendations (Promote better understanding of the approach and usefulness of "community-based participatory research models" and the importance of including prevention and intervention components in these models)

The Administrator should work through the Domestic Policy Council to establish an Interagency Task Force on Community-Based Participatory Health Research to provide better understanding of the principles of community-based participatory health research and to examine how to increase support, both moral and financial, for such research efforts. This Task Force should also deal with interagency cooperation (see "C" below).

- • *Rueben Warren, Agency for Toxic Substance and Disease Registry stated that partnering with communities to document environmental hazards and better data collection from communities will help to identify areas of need and help to improve methods on providing healthcare.* (HRS)

- *"...I personally would like to recommend that the NEJAC work to help enact or enforce existing policies that will make it mandatory for every agency that needs to be involved to foster partnerships with communities to develop corrective measures through a joint effort with any and all agency resources, such as DHHS, because there's so many different entities that come up under that Department of Health and Human Services, such as HRSA."* (Charlotte Keyes, II - 414)

The Interagency-Community Task Force on Community-Based Participatory Research should:

a. Develop a consensus definition of "community-based participatory health research." Recognizing the efforts that the National Institute of Environmental Health Sciences has made in community-based research, we recommend that their definition be used as a workbase.

b. Educate partners about appreciating and adapting to the "culture" of the community as well as appreciate and make use of the inherent capabilities within the communities.

- *"...I believe that there should be a remedial education project designed and developed with agency representatives from federal, state, and local communities with them in mind, involving community representation in the design of that educational project....."* (Donnell Wilkins, II - 471)

c. Implement strategies to learn to work with as well as improve the quality, understandability, and timeliness of communications with the community.

- *"We, as the CDC, need to spend a lot of time and effort on all the issues of communication, health communication, strategies, communication between communities and us, communication between the agencies. We need much more effort there, and I would recommend some focus on that."* (Michael Sage, II - 253)

- *"ORD needs to have a greater focus on getting information out to communities rather than just focus on research...* (HRS)

d. Always include a component for intervention and prevention in the community.

- *Expand and extend the funding of prevention/intervention partnerships "pilots" with impacted community organizations, grassroots groups, and minority academic institutions as th elead agencies.* (VII - 4)

- *Explore public/private (community, government, HMOs, etc.) health promotion and prevention/intervention models to address environmental health problems (i.e. childhood asthma). (VII - 4)*

e. There needs to be an examination of how existing funds can be redefined so it can be used for community-based participatory health research.

- *"...Some of the recommendations that I would make is that we need to encourage broad based -- I'm not using the word "funding" here as the focus -- but broad based funding for CDC and state and local departments, meaning funding that will allow us to deal with real public health concerns, real issues that people have, and not necessarily the narrow-focused funding that we have. We need to encourage -- once we have that broad based funding, we need to commit to program-specific projects to address environmental justice concerns, which we really have an inability to do at this time.* (Michael Sage, II - 253)

- *"...Go back to funding the CUP grants that were established years ago that provided the Community University Partnerships....."* (Robert Bullard, II - 69)

- *Regulatory agencies responsible of protecting people's health and environment need to secure funding to impacted communities to hire consultants to do health assessments/surveys and /or studies. (VII - 4)*

- *Explore models that utilize creative ways of financing prevention programs (i.e. fines and penalties levied against companies for violations can be designate(d) to community programs instead of going to general fund. (VII - 4)*

f. Provide substantial grant funding not only to institutions, but prioritize funding to well-established community organizations as the grant administrator to improve sustainability. The period of funding should be at least four years.

- *"I think that if you are a funding agency and you are trying to decide whether you should give out two-year grants at $250,000 a year or four-year grants at $50,000 to $100,000, I would go for the four-year grants....It's that ongoing consistent funding that's really most important."* (Patrick Kinney, II - 63)

- *Design environmental justice health research, education, and prevention/intervention RFPs/RFAs that call for partnerships research in which the community-based organization is an equal partner in the research endeavor. (VII - 4)*

g. Examine new approaches to funding these projects.

> *"I think that you might want to give some consideration to the idea with multiple sources from different Federal agencies to fund centers that are focused on specifically community-based participatory research, probably centers which are jointly run by community groups or research or clinical-oriented you know, health care organizations."* (Patrick Kinney, II - 64)

h. Implement a process by which granting institutions verify community participation beginning with the research proposal throughout the duration of the funding cycle.

> *"...It is incumbent upon funding agencies to verify partnerships, to insure that it is not some inequitable, patched together, kind of network. This effort requires the evaluation of whether a partnership described on paper, on a grant application, actually exists and will survive post-funding...."* (V - 6)

i. Reexamine how Federal environmental missions and resources are divided among agencies; especially as related to Indian country and Native Alaskan villages.

> *Because Federal environmental missions and resources are divided among and in some cases overlap between various agencies, coordinate and pool available technical and financial resources to provide environmental health-related services to Federally recognized tribes equitably, efficiently, and effectively. Towards this end, the Bureau of Indian Affairs, Environmental Protection Agency, Department of Housing and Urban Development, and the Indian Health Service should appraise the usefulness and implementation of the national MOU, previously discussed, and take appropriate steps to enhance and better promote interagency coordination and collaboration pertaining to the protection of health and the environment within Indian country and Alaska Native villages. The MOU 2000 may serve as a model for better implementing these efforts at regional and local Indian country and Alaska Native village levels.* (VI - 8)

j. Modify the standard peer review process to be more reflective of community-based participatory research products.

> *Expand pool of people of color and community-based organization leaders on review panels for research grants with compensation.* (VII - 4)

> *Expand definition of "experts" to include impacted residents.* (VII - 4)

II.B Translating Current and Future Scientific Knowledge Into Positive Action

II.B.1 Background

The transformation of laboratory-based (i.e., controlled) research to policy action is imperative. Today, there is likely both science and data held within various Federal agencies that is not being shared in a timely way and may result in both duplication of effort as well as less than optimum decisions.

- *"...I do believe that we need to address what is already existing in agencies and research the tools and resources that exist and encourage the continuance of interagency interaction between those entities. I believe that the answers that we're looking for already exist and there needs to be a push and a demand from this body to dig deeper into making certain that agencies are speaking with each other, sharing resources, and are talking to one another."* (Donnell Wilkins, II-472)

- *"scientific knowledge is not power unless it's applied."* (Jon Kerner, II - 244)

This section brings forth recommendations extracted primarily from the many public comments and panelists during the meeting that emphasized the need to use research as a tool for policy and service to the community. Many comments suggested that there has been a significant delay experienced in getting results to the community.

- *"...We have a lag time between the translation of science and its use in community education and prevention. A big issue for us. I would also hope that the Health and Research Subcommittee would kind of take a look at that issue and give us some of their concerns there and some suggestions."* (Michael Sage, II - 254)

II.B.2 Recommendations (Translating Current and Future Scientific Knowledge Into Positive Action)

The EPA Administrator should take a lead role in developing partnerships and collaborative projects among the traditional research-based entities (e.g., societies, association, universities) and more service-based institutions (e.g., Federal, state, local and tribal governments) in a goal to expand the channels for policy development and research dissemination and diffusion. Specifically, the Administrator should:

a. Ensure that EPA's research agendas are developed with consultation from various stakeholders groups by consulting with communities, Federally recognized tribes, and other stakeholders in the designing, planning, and implementing of environmental health research projects.

- *"As a community leader, I understand that the advisory panels or councils are the entities that lead the Agency to develop policies. The problem we are having is that these panels or councils do not have the appropriate community representation seated in the table, participating in the decision process. It's not a matter of communities acting as peer reviewers is a big part of the process. Communities are not properly represented in those panels."* (Ramos, II - 145)

b. Develop guidelines that emphasize the need to resolve existing problems, not just the need for further research.

- *"So it's not a matter of having the facts, having the science, having the data; it's a matter of whether or not we have the resolve and commitment to end this problem."* (Robert Bullard, II - 45-48)

- *Integrate environmental justice principles into the health research and health education programs, especially programs that service low-income and people of color communities.* (VII - 3)

c. Develop more mission-directed research or methods to ensure that the returns on the research investment can be applied to current policy and technical issues.

- *"One of the things that we recognized was that it was not only good enough for us to actually look at collecting this type of data with this new approach, but to also begin to use the data to help influence change, change that would make a lasting and significant impact in the quality of the lives in the communities which we serve. To that end, we have taken the data not only to be placed on shelves, but really taken it to the policymakers and presented it to them as we forged our demands for change in terms of the policies that impacted our air quality."* (Cecil Corbin-Mark, II - 315)

- *Design study to access possible regressive and discriminatory impact of health care practices on low-income and people of color.* (VII - 3)

- *Develop tools to identify and access impacts of environmental policies on low-income and people of color.* (VII - 3)

- *Design health research plans to include domestic, cross-border and international links.* (VII - 3)

d. Recruit citizens to participate in the design and execution of the research to be performed, and that communication during all phases of the research be open and reciprocal. Specifically, all collaborative research projects should have the following basic principles:

(1) Based on shared interest in the research that will be performed and provide each participant with meaningful (i.e., value-added) results.

(2) Establish a set of explicit outcome goals and procedures before collaboration begins.

(3) Establish a high level of trust and communication between participants.

- • *"As a community leader, I understand that the advisory panels or councils are the entities that lead the agency to develop policies. The problem we are having is that these panels or councils do not have the appropriate community representation seated in the table, participating in the decision process. It's not a matter of communities acting as peer reviewers is a big part of the process. Communities are not properly represented in those panels."* (Ramos, II - 145, VI - 6)

(4) Ensure that environmental health research data is reported back to tribal governments and communities promptly and in an understandable manner.

e. Where there are existing data gaps based on incomplete scientific data, commit sufficient resources to finding answers to these research questions that promise to lie at the heart of future policy decisions. However, in the light of existing data gaps, steps should be taken to address the current conditions of communities of concern.

- *"I think there's still value to research. However, I think we should take certain precautionary steps applying the precautionary principle to certain public policies where we reached those limits of science. It's important for us to stop and intervene in those problems that are happening in the community and understand that there is another principle out there that we from the environmental justice movement put forward. That's self-determination."* (Carlos Porras, II - 140)

- *"There's lots of information we don't have, lots of areas we don't have information on. But it's not just enough to say, "Well, we just don't know that." We have to pursue a strategy to talk about intervening and preventing environmental health hazards and environmental degradation."* (Robert Bullard, II - 55-56)

- *Document successful community-based research models and assess their applicability and generalizability to larger population.* (VII - 4)

f. Direct additional funding and resources to communities that deal with these problems environmental health problems on a daily basis.

- *"We've been hearing this for years that lead poisoning is a problem. We have statistics and facts that lead poisoning and asthma is a problem. We know this for a fact. We can do something about this, but it's not getting back to the community, to the problem. How can we change this? This is what I'm coming here to find out, what can we actually do and stop talking about doing? What can we do to get this information and funding and resources to the community, to the people who are actually involved with these problems."* (Bill Burns, I - 83)

g.   Whenever feasible, EPA should develop procedures that allow communities to conduct health surveys on their own communities and, to the extent possible, act as peer reviewers for certain studies.

- *"One of the things that we've done is that basically this health survey was conducted by actually the community, the affected community."* (Robert Bullard, II - 59).

- *"...Who are your peers? I mean, if they're community-based partners, you need community-based folks doing the review. And we know that. But then getting a common understanding between reviewers about what's good science and what's good community-based research is also a challenge."* (Jon Kerner, II-291-2)

h.   *Request that the Indian Health Service make its annual data on health status readily available to each Federally recognized tribe and other Federal agencies.* (VI - 9)

i.   Ensure that EPA sponsored research is driven in terms of how can research impact policy.

- *"I would say that be driven in terms of how can research impact policy. That may be a dirty word, but policy can drive a lot of this stuff. In many cases the only science involved in why Black and Latino children are being lead poisoned -- the only science is political science."* (Robert Bullard, II - 70)

j.   *Support innovative and sustainable technologies within Indian country and Alaska Native villages (e.g., waterless toilets, solar energy systems, and constructed wetlands).* (VI - 8)

k.   Develop a nationwide, baseline tracking of priority diseases - asthma and chronic respiratory diseases; birth defects; developmental disorders; cancers, especially childhood cancers; and neurological diseases, such as Alzheimer's, multiple sclerosis and Parkinson's - and priority exposures, such as PCBs and dioxin; heavy metals, such as mercury and lead; pesticides; water and air contaminants. A tracking system specifically targeting school children should be part of this effort.

- *"...We agreed to prepare a resolution for approval, recommending that EPA establish and effective national facility registry system for all operating facilities that emit hazardous chemicals, and make the information accessible and understandable to the public."* (Marinelle Payton, IV - 188)

- *America's Environmental Health Gap: Why the Nation Needs a Nationwide Health Tracking Network,* The Pew Environmental Health Commission, September 2000 (http://pewenvirohealth.jhsph.edu/html/reports/pewpressrelease.pdf)

- *Every public school in the United States should have a disease registry to identify health care needs of children* (VII - 3)

l. Develop an Agency strategy to discuss intervening and preventing environmental hazards and environmental degradation in disproportionately impacted communities.

- *"We have to pursue a strategy to talk about intervening and preventing environmental health hazards and environmental degradation."* (Robert Bullard, II - 55-56) *EPA must translate research into intervention.*

- *"We define translational research as a conversion of finding from basic, clinical or epidemiological environmental science research into information, resources or tools that can be applied by health care providers and community residents to improve public health outcome in at-risk populations."* (Charles Wells, II - 233)

- *Regulatory agencies should emphasis precaution and prevention instead of just regulatory action.* (VII - 3)

m. Emphasize that the scientific approach should be in balance with the recognition that the community must play an increasingly active role in decisions about research and public health intervention.

- *"...You don't necessarily have to uncover all things that need to be uncovered in research to do something about it because essentially more research often leads to more unanswered questions. So, from my own personal standpoint it is necessary to implement intervention programs, those that we may call mitigation programs."* (Hilary Inyang, II - 182)

n. Complete the development of the "Cumulative Risk Framework" and then a Cumulative Risk Guideline, to be used by the Agency in assessing potential EJ communities.

- *"Today I'd like to talk about a process that EPA has to ultimately establish some guidelines for doing cumulative risk assessments. We have other guidelines in the agency; we have guidelines for cancer assessment, guidelines for exposure assessment.*

The guidelines for cumulative risk assessment will be another of these sets of documents that kind of outlines to the agency what it should and should not be doing when we're doing these sorts of scientific endeavors." (Michael Callahan II - 200)

II.C   More Effective Interagency Collaboration and Cooperation

II.C.1   Background

More and more, as we look at solving the myriad of problems facing our most beleaguered communities, we find that no one agency can possibly deal with the range of issues that need confronting:

- *"... A lot of energies are targeted at EPA, but EPA cannot do it all. That means that we have to have interagency cooperation and collaboration. We have to work across the board to talk about how to get all these folks to the table. So this is very good when we talk about having it at the various agencies. Not just the Federal government, but also state agencies, local health departments, state health departments, and county health departments, et cetera, work on these issues."* (Robert Bullard, II - 53)

- *"......that this research that happens needs to be multi-disciplinary, multi-agency; that the Federal agencies do need to work together in focusing on these environmental justice communities, these sites, where a lot of work has been done and continues to be done."* (Katsi Cook, II - 109)

- *"...We need to work with other agencies to come up with holistic solutions. You know, oftentimes people do what they think they can do in terms of government agencies, but people in communities just see that as a very narrow kind of solution. We really need to think of holistically how to help people and how we can fit into maybe broader solutions that will help people."* (Henry Falk II - 216)

- *"I think that there is in fact a stovepiping across Federal agencies. It is not uncommon for people to believe that environmental justice is an issue for EPA and the other agencies, when they sit at the table, are doing us a favor...Well, in fact, the environment is a factor for every agency. Health is a factor for every agency."* (Hal Zenick, II - 267)

- *"We need to work together to build a unified system to support community needs."* (HRS)

- *An academician stated that these agencies have tunnel vision, and should attempt to develop an integrated plan to attack health disparities.* (V - 14)

II.C.2 Recommendations (More Effective Interagency Collaboration and Cooperation)

The Administrator should request that the Interagency Task Force, recommended in (A) earlier in this document, determine how they can work together to better serve beleaguered EJ communities and eliminate health disparities. Some of the issues may be able to be dealt with through the Interagency Work Group EJ Action Agenda.

- *"The aim of the EJ Action Agenda is to bring together the resources of 11 Federal agencies to help environmentally and economically distressed communities. Together, 11 Federal agencies and departments, identified 15 environmental justice demonstration projects. The anticipated result will be to use Federal resources in a targeted way to improve life in 15 minority and low-income communities that suffer disproportionate environmental impacts. Based on our experience with these pilot projects, we'll try to add more projects and broaden agency participation in the future."* (Michael McCabe, II - 153)

a. *Direct the Interagency Working Group on Environmental Justice, in collaboration with Federally recognized tribes, to use its Roundtable on Environmental Justice in Indian Country as a model or vehicle for identifying possible strategies to address unmet environmental health and research needs in Indian country and Alaska Native villages promptly, effectively, and equitably.* (VI-4)

b. Either the IWG or the proposed Interagency Task Force should determine how to properly involve the Department of Education, as a partner, in solving those issues identified with school children and schools.

- *"So when we talk about childhood lead poisoning, it is not only a health problem, it's an environmental problem because lead is an environmental issue, and it's an educational problem -- we're talking about learning disabilities. So when we're talking about solving the problem of lead poisoning, we just can't be going to the EPA. The Department of Education needs to be involved, the Department of Housing and Urban Development needs to be involved."* (Robert Bullard II - 53)

- *We are also looking at children that are attending schools on contaminated sites. There tends to be more -- it looks like there's more and more of a trend toward locating schools on contaminated sites. These children need to be studied because hopefully this won't continue very long and we won't have the opportunity to study these children right now. We believe that the environmental exposure in air and soil should be looked at.* (Mark Mitchell II-451)

c. The IWG should work to ensure that the Department of Transportation is engaged and has access to assistance from environmental/health related agencies in dealing with transportation related issues that may be causing disparities.

- *"....I suggest to you that there are other issues, and there are other major issues. These issues include geographic location and infrastructure of the community, the condition of roadways -- and I'm so pleased that we have a representative from the Department of Transportation here today."* (Michael Rathsom, II - 261)

d. The proposed Interagency Task Force should develop a mechanism to establish responsibilities and measure accountability for the agencies that should be engaged in eliminating health disparities.

- *"We need to bring the all these agencies that are supposed to be at the table......Where is the accountability of all these agencies that should be at the table today?...We need to have them at the table now."* (Rose Augustine, II - 72)

Recommendations **II.A.2 - e, g, and i** above, are also appropriate for "More Effective Interagency Collaboration and Cooperation."

II.D Including Socioeconomic and Cultural Factors in Health Assessments

II.D.1 Background

The overwhelming consensus in pre-meeting interviews was that all socioeconomic and cultural factors (SES) are important in addressing community health concerns.

- *"...for more than 800 years..... people have known that higher rates of death, illness, and disability have tended to concentrate in the poorest members of the community."* (Walter Handy, II - 196)

These factors include social, behavioral, economic, cultural, political issues and traditional values and practices. It is the general consensus of stakeholders that ample evidence exists of a relationship between socioeconomic and /or cultural factors and health impacts and are important contributors to health disparities. (V - 12)

A number of stakeholders spoke to the types of socioeconomic and cultural factors that should be considered:

- *... socioeconomic conditions and health, absolute and relative poverty, standard of living, access to healthy foods, position at work (occupational environment), are all factors relevant to health...* (V - 12)

- *...consideration and attention need to be directed at the role of other factors, such as psychological stressors (i.e., job security, safety issues, housing, etc.), class, outside stressors, environmental stressors, economic and racial segregation and others, may play in relation to health disparities.* (Samara Swanston, II-187-8)

- *"...if you are talking about environmental justice, you must discuss issues of class in relation to race, gender, and other factors. This should include informed social scientist' input, not just physical science..."* (Samara Swanston, II-194)

- *"The vulnerabilities and susceptibilities of children to these environmental attacks."* (Carlos Porras, II-104)

- *"The measures most commonly used to evaluate socioeconomic status are income, education and occupational prestige. These measures are limited in that they do not capture significant components of social stratification than can influence health status. Other measures of socioeconomic status include the conditions in which an individual lives, intergenerational transfers of wealth since inheritance of wealth occurs less frequently among minorities, and a consideration of socioeconomic status in this country must also include race because socioeconomic status is transformed by racism."* (Samara Swanston, II-187-8)

- *"Social support and coping style may also offer keys to examining the more difficult social contexts of health status."* (Walter Handy, II-197)

- *Social and cultural disruption of traditional Native societies, lack of education and economic opportunities, and high levels of unemployment and poverty. These all put Indian people at higher risk. Disparities in health are aggravated by a disparity of resources, especially the gap in health care spending for Indian people compared to other Americans."* (Michael Rathsom, II-257)

- *Cultural barriers, as well as language barriers, need to be included in socioeconomic status. Race, gender, location of residence, location of workplace and cultural distinction are measures that need to be included in SES because SES does not mean the same thing in communities of color than it does in white communities."* (Samara Swanston, II-194)

There is a considerable body of evidence, that socioeconomic factors are linked to observed health disparities. Some specific examples where sited by a panel member:

- *"most people are aware of the many studies demonstrating that even after adjustment for insurance and clinical status, similarly situated minorities are less likely to receive coronary angioplasty bypass surgery, angioplasty, hemodialysis, kidney transplants, intensive care for pneumonia, and other aggressive disease treatment. Racism even directly affects health status since in several studies an association has been established between reported racial discrimination and hypertension. So, income, education and occupational prestige measures do not measure the same thing in our community. SES affects or influences health care. According to cancer experts, socioeconomic status plays a role in the use of different screening tests and higher SES is correlated with greater use of screening tests, more aggressive therapy and a greater chance for cancer survival. Socioeconomic status plays a role in obesity, leading to diabetes. Diabetes, for example, was virtually nonexistent among Native Americans until many Native Americans were forced to change their traditional diet due to the effects of pollution and also forced relocations away from reservations. Now Native Americans have the highest diabetes rate in the United States."* (Samara Swanston, II-194)

Several stakeholders observed the need to examine each community individually, because the potential difference in socioeconomic and cultural factors affecting health outcomes are significant.

- *"SES does not have the same meaning in communities of color as it does in other communities."* (V - 12)

- *American Indians/Alaska Natives (AI/AN) are particularly susceptible to health impacts from pollution due to their traditional and cultural uses of natural resources and, in fact, AI/AN "have greater exposure risks than the general population as a result of their dietary practices and unique cultures that embrace the environment." Fishing, hunting, and gathering often are part of a spiritual, cultural, social, and economic lifestyle, and the survival of many AI/ANs depends on subsistence hunting, fishing, and gathering. In some instances, the right to engage in these activities is legally protected by treaty. Additionally, many AI/ANs also use water, plants, and animals in their traditional and religious practices and ceremonies. As a result, contamination of the water, soil, plants, and animals and the subsequent accumulation of these contaminants in the people through ingestion and contact not only endangers the health of AI/ANs, but also threatens the well-being of their future generations and undermines the cultural survival of tribes and Alaska Native villages.* (VI - 3-4)

Throughout the interviews and meeting, there were many calls for more and better research and data:

- *These are data gaps, very real data gaps."* (Carlos Porras, II-104)

- *I think that an overall conclusion of this committee is not only the fact that there is a need for greater research, particularly research that understands and links the relationship between environmental causes of disease and health disparities in minority low income communities, but that this kind of research needs to be done in a different way."* (Charles Lee, II- 34)

- *......although health data is collected by race and ethnicity, there are no indicators of social class on the birth certificate, no information on income, health insurance, etc. This makes it difficult to determine the impact of race versus socioeconomic status when examining health effects.* (V - 11)

A social scientist (Roger Kasperson, Executive Director of the Stockholm Environment Institute and EPA Science Advisory Board member) gives us a more focused definition for vulnerability. Social science looks at vulnerability as being made up of four things:

(1) susceptibility or sensitivity (which is a different or more pronounced dose-response);

(2) differential exposure (including historical exposure, body burden, background exposure, etc.);

(3) differential preparedness to withstand the insult of the stressor; and (4) differential ability to recover from the effects of the stressor. He said that in the social science literature, "vulnerability" was linked to what kind of coping systems and resources a community has.

II.D.2 Recommendations (Including Socioeconomic and Cultural Factors in Health Assessments)

____The EPA Administrator should support EPA and other Federal agencies efforts to include socioeconomic and cultural factors when doing health assessments, as well as intervention and prevention programs. These efforts should include the following:

a. Consider how socioeconomic and cultural factors may affect the nature of intervention/prevention options <u>and</u> how these factors impact the acceptability of those options to the community.

- *Such options should be based not only on science, but also should address and incorporate the traditional knowledge of a community. For example, limitations on the consumption of traditional foods due to pollution danger may trigger unique social, economic, and health problems within AI/AN communities.* (VI-9)

> • *Design methodologies to access community impacts)environmental, human health, socioeconomic, cultural, etc.) existing burdens (multiple and cumulative impacts), and "vulnerable" populations (low-income, children, elderly, workers, women, etc.) (VII - 4)*

b. Establish an interagency committee to foster and coordinate research and data collection on the impact of socioeconomic and cultural factors on health disparities.

> • *"...the ability to effectively ensure healthy communities is absolutely dependent upon us being able to take a more integrated approach to looking at the dynamics between those factors. I think that there is in fact a stove piping across Federal agencies. It is not uncommon for people to believe that environmental justice is an issue for EPA and the other agencies, when they sit at the table, are doing us a favor...Well, in fact, the environment is a factor for every agency. Health is a factor for every agency."* (Hal Zenick, II-267)

c. Agencies need to train and/or hire additional social scientists and assign them to work on community-based assessments.

> • *....scientists from the social sciences (sociology, psychology, behavioral sciences, anthropology, psychometrics, etc.) should be included in research activities. The community model would benefit from social science. They have a great deal to offer in the area of social behavior, psychological stress etc. (V - 8)*

d. As part of examining prevention/intervention strategies, social support mechanisms and strategies for helping the community to cope, should be included.

> • *......identify effective coping strategies and social support mechanisms among other community residents.* (Walter Handy, II-197)

e. Ensure that agency staff and managers have a thorough understanding of Federal Indian law and policies, tribal culture, and the unique governmental structure of Federally recognized Indian tribes, including Alaska Native villages. This is particularly important for those people directly working on these issues. (VI - 13)

II.E   Responding to the Urgent Needs of Medically Underserved Communities

   II.E.1   Background

The primary object of this theme is to recommend to the Administrator methods for linking members of a community (i.e., individuals directly affected by adverse environmental conditions), with researchers, policy makers, health care providers and educators in an objective to find solutions for their existing health-related problems.

Development of community-based strategies to address environmental health problems requires approaches that are not typically familiar to the research and medical communities. The distinctive needs of individual communities and their inhabitants are rarely considered in identifying environmental health problems and devising appropriate medical intervention.

II.E.2 Recommendations (Responding to the Urgent Needs of Medically Underserved Communities)

These recommendations are designed to encourage EPA and the member agencies of the proposed Interagency Task Force on Community-Based Participatory Health Research to aggressively participate in the development of new modes of communication and to ensure that community organizations actively participant with policy makers, researchers and health care providers in developing responses and setting priorities for intervention and mitigation strategies. Specifically, the Administrator should:

a. Encourage the development of high-quality, audience-appropriate information and support services for specific health problems (e.g., asthma) and health-related decisions for all segments of the population, especially under served persons.

b. Encourage the development of more community health centers, as authorized by the Public Health Service Act of 1975, to provide comprehensive primary medical care and preventive health services.

- *"We also need health facilities. We need health care for these people who doctors are still pondering what their ailments are; they're treating them for whatever they could possibly come up with a name for."* (David Baker, II-429)

- *Health care should be a right regardless of income status everyone should have access to adequate, quality and accessible health care.* (VII - 4)

c. Participate in more comprehensive community-based programs that provide more hands on tactics (e.g, home visits).

- *"I would suggest that one of the things that we might want to consider is how do we begin to combine our expertise that when we look at a community we can begin to understand what are some of the things that in a community partnership we can begin to treat, even if it's the symptoms, that begin to improve the health of the community as we try and understand what those triggers are. There's a variety of approaches. One of the things I would offer in terms of whether this is realistic is perhaps we can center on a limited number of communities over the next three to four years, develop -- I hate the word, but develop a swat team type of mentality. Can we go in with a group of experts working with the community and local folks, do the diagnostic, try and determine where can we influence, persuade, implement some changes in the conditions in that community, and then step back and make some assessment of have we been successful, what were the barriers, and I think critically when I have to go back to my agency and talk about this -- it is, and what are the constraints."* (Hal Zenick, II-271)

d. ••Develop a nationwide, baseline tracking of priority diseases - asthma and chronic respiratory diseases; birth defects; developmental disorders; cancers, especially childhood cancers; and neurological diseases, such as Alzheimer's, multiple sclerosis and Parkinson's - and priority exposures, such as PCBs and dioxin; heavy metals, such as mercury and lead; pesticides; water and air contaminants.

- •• *"...We agreed to prepare a resolution for approval, recommending that EPA establish and effective national facility registry system for all operating facilities that emit hazardous chemicals, and make the information accessible and understandable to the public."* (Marinelle Payton, IV-188)

- •• *America's Environmental Health Gap: Why the Nation Needs a Nationwide Health Tracking Network,* The Pew Environmental Health Commission, September 2000 (http://pewenvirohealth.jhsph.edu/html/reports/pewpressrelease.pdf)

e. Participate in research in identifying and interpreting national trends and issues relative to the health status of persons disproportionately effected by environmental hazards.

f. Develop, promote and participate in efforts to improve the management, operational effectiveness, and efficiency of health care systems and facilities in minority and low-income communities.

g. *Stress the importance of facilitating and assisting Indian tribes in coordinating health planning, in obtaining and utilizing health resources available through Federal, State and local programs in operating comprehensive health programs.* (VI - 8)

h. *Support legislative initiatives, including but not limited to the reauthorization of the Indian Health Care Improvement Act, that will eliminate inequities in Federal funding to address the alarmingly high levels of unmet environmental and health needs of AI/ANs, regardless of where they live.* (VI - 8)

i. *Assert a leadership role among Federal agencies in developing new financing mechanisms and leveraging all available resources to fund and implement environmental health-related projects and research in Indian country and Alaska Native villages.* (VI - 8)

j. Establish a Pollution Victims Compensation Fund designed to do the following:
(a) pay the health care costs of pollution victims; (b) provide technical assistance to community in holding responsible corporations accountable for containing and cleaning up uncontrolled toxic sites; (c) provide tax incentives to industries to retool production processes to reduce toxic discharges; and (d) retain job placement and worker transition costs associated with displacement created by production process changes motivated by pollution prevention efforts. (Jackie Ward, I - 135)

k. Support educational efforts directed at health professionals to be better trained on environmental justice issues. Specifically, medical students and residents should be better trained in environmental and occupational medicine. These individuals should attend toxic health training courses and become aware of how to treat environmentally related diseases as they relate to short-term and long-term exposure.

- *"The third bullet is one I've mentioned and I think that without this commitment we're not going to make very much progress. And that is, I believe it is absolutely essential that the public health and the medical community, which is a major powerful player in this country, recognizes that environmental conditions are a major etiological factor in health status."* (Hal Zenick, II-267)

- *"I also recommend that existing and new physicians, nurses, and other medical professionals go through toxic health training to become aware on how to service the needs of these environmental diseases as they relate to short-term and long-term exposure."* (Charlottee Keys, II-415)

- *All health care workers should receive training on environmental health.* (VII - 3)

l. Develop initiatives that focus on addressing environmental primary health care needs through utilizing existing assessments and medical and financial support that you already have to address intervention and prevention.

- *".. I also recommend that we stop talking about environmental diseases and begin to focus on addressing environmental primary health care needs through utilizing existing assessment and use the medical and financial support that you already have to address intervention and prevention through medical testing and medical referrals and prevent diseases through not using funds to place communities at risk close to poison sites and in workplaces that poison humans to death."* (Charlottee Keys, II-415)

m. Work with state, local and tribal health officials, community representatives, and other Federal agencies to improve health and environmental surveillance and monitoring activities in minority and low-income populations disproportionately impacted by high and adverse environmental exposures.

n. Expand the existing relationship with the Agency for Toxic Substances Disease Registry (ATSDR) to providing funding for health care facilities at national priority list sites and at Federal facilities where environmental contamination is effecting the public health.

o. *"Therefore, we also recommend that this committee recommend to EPA -- that NEJAC recommend to EPA that they expand their relationship with the Agency for Toxic Substances Disease Registry and provide funding for health care facilities at national priority list sites and at Federal facilities where radiation and all kinds of other chemicals used by the military in warfare have been stored and are now killing people who are associated with that facility."* (Marvin Crafter, I-64-65)

p. Establish a program to prevent the future siting of schools on contaminated property and increase efforts to examine existing schools sited on contaminated sites or located in heavily polluted areas.

- *"We have five schools less than a mile from these facilities on the west end. If we go to the east end, we have six, a high school, junior high, and K through 5 and nurseries. And they even live closer than that.* (Mr. Mouton III - 26)

- *"We are also looking at children that are attending schools on contaminated sites. There tends to be more -- it looks like there's more and more of a trend toward locating schools on contaminated sites. These children need to be studied because hopefully this won't continue very long and we won't have the opportunity to study these children right now. We believe that the environmental exposure in air and soil should be looked at."* (Mark Mitchell II - 451)

- *We are leveraging an EPA study and hope to do personal exposure research on the students in a school district in Houston which is downwind of some major source. We hope to get a handle there in a good statistically sound peer-reviewed way of the kinds of exacerbation of asthma that could result from exposure to air toxics.* (Ray Campion II - 129)

III. Appendices

III.A Recommendations Work Group

Rose M. Augustine
President, Tucsonans for A Clean Environment

Henry Falk
Assistant Administrator, Agency for Toxic Substances and Disease Registry

Jon F. Kerner
Assistant Deputy Director, Division of Cancer Control and Population Sciences
National Cancer Institute, National Institutes of Health

Lillian Mood RN
Community Liaison, South Carolina Department of Health and Environmental Control

Marinelle Payton, Chair
Chair, Dept. of Public Health
Jackson State, School of Allied Health Sciences

Carlos Porras
Communities for a Better Environment

William Sanders
EPA, Director, Office of Pollution Prevention and Toxics

Michael Sage
National Center for Environmental Health
Centers for Disease Control and Prevention National

Peggy M Shepard
Executive Director, West Harlem Environmental Action Inc

Jane Stahl
Deputy Assistant Commissioner, Connecticut Department of Environmental Protection

Charles Wells
Office of the Director, National Institute of Environmental Health Sciences

Pat Wood
Senior Manager, Federal Regulatory Affairs
Georgia Pacific Corporation

Hal Zenick
EPA, Associate Director, National Health and Environmental Effects Research Laboratory

III.B   May 2000 NEJAC HEALTH AND RESEARCH SUBCOMMITTEE Meeting Synopsis

The Health and Research Subcommittee of the National Environmental Justice Advisory Council (NEJAC) conducted a one-day meeting on Thursday, May 25, 2000, during a four-day meeting of the NEJAC in Atlanta, Georgia. Members of the Health and Research Subcommittee engaged in dialogue with representatives of an Interagency Forum (Theme: "Healthcare: Establishing Partnerships with Minorities, Tribal, and Low-Income Communities"):

William H. Sanders III, Director, Office of Pollution Prevention and Toxics, (OPPT) U.S. Environmental Protection Agency (EPA), began the Interagency Forum discussion with opening remarks on some initial observations he made regarding the panel session the day before. He observed that we are trying to fit the problem into the existing scientific structure, rather than fit the science with the problem and we need to better manage public expectations. Government is too slow and we take too long to do something. We need to improve the conditions that affect public health and not just study and move before the dead bodies show up. If we proceed with the status quo (random samples, court challenge, and peer review), it would take a long time before anything will get done. Rather than talking about research, look at action - one area is looking beyond compliance and to work with industry to get them to be cleaner in the first place, e.g., OPPT's voluntary programs.

Henry Falk, Assistant Administrator, Agency for Toxic Substances and Disease Registry (ATSDR), stated that whatever efforts take place, they need to be sustainable. Types of partnerships that need to be created might need to be broader - to include education, etc. Try to organize recommendations in different levels: 1) Community levels: include universities, and local and state health departments; collect data on diseases; 2) Federal level: agencies need to work together better; and 3) Systemic level: think broadly and look for a systemic solution to the problem. ATSDR's priority areas of research include documentation of environmental hazards; better data on disease frequency related to the environment. Improve methods in working with diverse groups to collect information.

Richard Gragg, Associate Director, Environmental Sciences Institute, Center for Environmental Justice and Equity, Florida A&M University, stated that communities have a distrust of federal and local government. Universities can often play the intermediary role, the role of educator for communities, facilitate between federal and state agencies, and look at problems in different ways, e.g., is health only physical health, or does it encompass more than that? He suggested that we need an inventory of communities and a framework for assessment.

John Kerner, Assistant Deputy Director, Research Dissemination and Diffusion, Division of Cancer Control and Population Sciences, National Cancer Institute (NCI), National Institute of Health, stated that science is only a tool, the question should be how can we best apply science to the Environmental Justice situation? We need: 1) a better relationship between university healthcare institutions and communities and to build links between the research and service delivery agencies, so that once the problems have been identified, there are resources to solve the issue; 2) good needs assessment at the community level (NCI is trying to develop tools to look at data at the county level, looking at unequal burdens between communities, and look at environmental and other factors); 3) What is the best prevention or intervention solution that Science tells us? 4) What infrastructure is available to take that intervention to the community?

Rebecca Lee-Pethel, National Center for Environmental Health (NCEH), Center for Disease Control, stated that Promotoras de Salud (health promoter) is a good concept and that some states have adopted its use for communities. NCEH is looking at communities that have used this program and how it can benefit others.

Francisco Tomei, Agency for Toxic Substances and Disease Registry, noted that federal agencies are involved in many activities and services. We need to work together to build a unified system to support community needs.

Reuben Warren, Agency for Toxic Substances and Disease Registry stated that partnering with communities to document environmental hazards and better data collection from communities will help to identify areas of need and help to improve methods on providing healthcare.

Charles Wells, Director, Environmental Health Sciences, National Institute of Environmental Health

Sciences (NIEHS), National Institute of Health, stated that NIEHS has been sponsoring community-based grants for partnering communities and academic. More grants structured toward healthcare are needed.

Jeannine Willis, Minority Health Office, Health Resource Services Administration (HRSA), Department of Health and Human Resources noted that HRSA and ATSDR have training partnerships so that primary healthcare providers can be trained to recognize symptoms from environmental hazards.

Harold Zenick, Acting Deputy Assistant Administrator for Science, Office of Research and Development (ORD), U.S. Environmental Protection Agency. ORD addresses this issue in three ways: 1) providing grants to community; 2) intramural taskforce: when Agency priorities links to Environmental Justice communities, there s opportunity to work with communities; 3) building stronger relationships with Regions. ORD needs to have a greater focus on getting information out to communities rather than just focus on research and should have a multi-media approach to identify source of contamination. Children are a central theme for ORD's exposure work. Also forming an interagency group would be most beneficial to look at human exposure

Summary of the Subcommittee Meeting

During the one-day meeting, members of the subcommittee discussed the following issues.

As a result of discussions by the subcommittee at the December 1999 NEJAC meeting, the subcommittee had an Interagency Forum to discuss building collaborations between agencies and communities to address healthcare issues. The Interagency Forum discussions included the role of each agency, priority areas of research, and a strategic plan to consider the next steps toward improving public health; implementation, development, and evaluation of future community-based health assessment; and pollution prevention and intervention issues in minority and low-income communities.

Also, members of the subcommittee and invited guests discussed at length a resolution to request that NEJAC establish a work group within the subcommittee to focus on the development of a strategic, Interagency Public Health Work Group.

In response to continued concerns expressed during public comment periods of the NEJAC, members of the subcommittee discussed a resolution recommending that the next NEJAC meeting focus on the issue of environmental justice arising from federal facilities in environmental compliance and remediation. In addition, it was agreed that the subcommittee include in the resolution that EPA prepare and submit for signature by President Clinton an Executive Order requiring that all federal agencies ensure compliance with EPA or state standards, whichever stricter, regarding site remediation, pollution control and abatement at all federal facilities, active or inactive, and further authorize EPA to monitor and enforce federal agency compliance with all environmental laws and standards.

Members of the subcommittee voted and established a Health and Research Subcommittee Work Group on Federal Facilities. The subcommittee will invite members of other subcommittees of the NEJAC, environmental justice community representatives, and EPA Federal Facility Enforcement Office and ATSDR's Office of Federal Facilities to participate in the Work Group.
Members of the subcommittee also agreed to prepare for consideration by the NEJAC a proposed resolution to make recommendations to EPA for improvement of community right-to-know laws.

Members of the Community Health Assessment Work Group of the subcommittee presented a report on their evaluation of the Decision Tree Model for Community-driven Environmental Health Assessment. Dr. Marinelle Payton, Harvard Medical School and Chair of the Health and Research Subcommittee, provided an overview of the Decision Tree Framework and plans for its future development in the coming year that will include incorporating the recommendations made by the Work Group.

Members of the subcommittee agreed to prepare for consideration by the Executive Council of the NEJAC a proposed resolution to make recommendations to EPA for the future development of the decision tree model as a priority for EPA.

As a result of the request by Mr. Damu Smith, GreenPeace, to Dr. Marinelle Payton, for the subcommittee to consider the Mossville Dioxin Exposure Assessment Study in Mossville, LA, the subcommittee had a joint session with the Waste and Facility Siting Subcommittee. The Joint session consisted of representatives from Mossville Environmental Action Now, GreenPeace, Louisiana Department of Health and Hospitals, ATSDR, and EPA Region 6. The purpose of the discussion was to consider the next steps of the exposure assessment study, to determine how to facilitate community participation, and how to utilize the information learned from this study to impact the nation.

Federal and state representatives agreed to work with the community to formulate a plan to further investigate the dioxin exposure assessment study in Mossville, LA and neighboring communities.

Significant Action Items and Proposed Resolutions

Following is a list of significant action items the members adopted during the subcommittee meeting:

Voted to establish an Interagency Work Group on Public Health which will include Health and Research Subcommittee members and invited representatives of the Interagency Forum to focus on developing a strategic plan to implement an integrated, collaborative, community-based public health agenda.

Develop a resolution that recommends to the Executive Council of the NEJAC that the next NEJAC meeting focus on the issue of environmental justice arising from federal facilities in environmental compliance and remediation. In addition, the resolution recommends EPA prepare and submit for signature by President Clinton an Executive Order requiring that all federal agencies ensure compliance with EPA or state standards, whichever stricter, regarding site remediation, pollution control and abatement of all federal facilities, active or inactive, and further authorize EPA to monitor and enforce federal agency compliance with all environmental laws and standards.

Adopt the recommendations from the Work Group on Community Environmental Health Assessment. The recommendations include (1) proposing a resolution to NEJAC that recommends that EPA support the Decision Tree Model as a priority issue, and (2) extending the terms of the workgroup and the Chair of the Subcommittee to maintain continuity of the development of the Decision Tree.

Voted to establish a Work Group on Federal Facilities. The subcommittee agreed to invite members of other subcommittees of the NEJAC, environmental justice community representatives, and EPA Federal Facility Enforcement Office and ATSDR's Office of Federal Facilities to participate in the Work Group.

Develop a resolution that the NEJAC recommends that EPA include criteria in the agency permitting processes to protect communities with comparatively poor health from additional pollution-releasing facilities.

Develop a resolution that the NEJAC recommends that EPA should establish an effective national facility registration system for all operating facilities that emit toxic chemicals and make information accessible and understandable to the public.

Develop a resolution that the NEJAC recommends that EPA support formation of a NEJAC Work Group on the Mossville Dioxin Exposure Assessment Study.

III.C A Synopsis of Stakeholder Representatives' Views Regarding Community-Based
Health Research Models Report, May 15, 2000 (V)

Synopsis of Stakeholder Representatives' Views Regarding Community-Based Health Research Models

A Preliminary Report
Prepared for the U.S. Environmental Protection Agency
Office of Environmental Justice
By
Adrienne L. Hollis, Ph.D.
Florida A&M University
Institute of Public Health

Table of Contents

Introduction..	1
Purpose of NEJAC Meeting...	3
Purpose of Stakeholder Interviews..	4
Description of Stakeholders and Interview Process......................................	4
Results - Themes and Accompanying Comments...	5-15
1. Developing Effective Partnerships...	5
2. Intervention and Prevention Activities..	6
3. Community-Based Research..	7
4. Current Models of Community-Based Research................................	10
5. Barriers and Data Gaps and Their Relationship to Health Effects......	11
6. Socioeconomic Vulnerabilities and Cultural Factors........................	12
7. Effective Risk Communication..	13
8. Sustainability...	14
9. Federal Agencies as Partners...	14
10. Other Stakeholder Comments...	15
Appendices	
A. List of Stakeholder Interviewees..	16
B. List of Interview Questions..	19
C. Models of Community-Based Research..	23

SUMMARY OF STAKEHOLDER INTERVIEWS

Introduction

Protecting the health of all communities represents a formidable challenge for the Environmental Protection Agency (EPA). According to the 1997 Strategic Plan, the mission of the U.S. Environmental Protection Agency is to protect human health and to safeguard the natural environment air, water, and land upon which life depends for all Americans. EPA must carry out this mission consistent with Executive Order 12898 on environmental justice, and existing protective environmental laws.

The Surgeon General of the Department of Health and Human Services issued in January 2000 the publication, "Healthy People 2010 Understanding and Improving Health." The second goal of Healthy People 2010 is to eliminate health disparities among different segments of the population, including differences that occur by race or ethnicity, education or income. These disparities are especially apparent in minority, low-income, and/or indigenous communities. Many of these same communities bear a disproportionate exposure to environmental pollutants that may underlie and/or contribute to these disparities. When such exposures are combined with other social and physical living conditions present in these environments, the potential for health disparities is magnified even further.

The Office of Environmental Justice requested the National Environmental Justice Advisory Council (NEJAC) to focus its attention on federal efforts to secure disease prevention and health improvement in communities where health disparities exist that may result from, or be exacerbated by, disproportionate effects of environmental pollutants and certain socioeconomic or cultural factors. This report presents the results of interviews with twenty-one (21) stakeholders drawn from government, academia, industry and community organizations.

The stakeholders interviewed here, though from a variety of backgrounds, shared some common beliefs and expectations. Everyone supported the need for developing an integrated model to address community-based health needs. They believed that assessment, intervention and prevention are three major components of a community-based health model. Most emphasized the need for an evaluation component to that model. This is a dynamic model, which requires concerted efforts not just by EPA but by many other federal departments and agencies. Responding appropriately to the multi-agency public health concerns of communities requires a multi-faceted response. Moreover, it was noted that a static definition of health is a barrier to disease prevention and health improvement. Health is not merely an outcome, but a proactive process that lead to an outcome.

A central theme which emerged from the interviews was a need for partnerships. There was strong focus on the issue of working with communities. All stakeholders were emphatic that actions be conducted in the community with having the community as an equal partner. In fact, there was unanimous agreement that the community, or a community-based organization, is the most critical component of a successful partnership. This theme is a critical element to the success of a community-based public health model. Going beyond the notion of research done "in or to" a community to research that "works with" a community is viewed as a critical link for translating assessment efforts into needed intervention and prevention activities.

There was strong support on the part of all interviewees for the concept of community-based health research models. Given the central role of community-based organizations, community-based research is, thus, an absolutely essential element of any successful federal effort to achieving an integrated community model that includes health assessment, intervention and prevention. Interviewees were able to identify many such successful partnerships. They point to the support of such partnership models by federal agencies, in particular, the National Institute for Environmental Health Sciences. There was general consensus that an evaluation of existing models would provide valuable information, as well as specific tools which can be adapted for specific projects.

There also existed uniformity of opinion that federal agencies must learn to better partner with each other. Currently, there is a prevailing impression among all stakeholders that federal agencies are working in an isolated manner. This was seen as a requisite condition for better partnerships with community and other stakeholders. A number of federal agencies were identified as potential partners in a community-based health research model. These included not only EPA and public health agencies but also agencies such as the Department of Transportation, Department of Energy, Department of Housing and Urban Development, Department of Agriculture, Department of Labor and others.

Special attention should be given to overcoming specific barriers to success of such community-based health research models. One such barrier is the need to capacity building for community- based organizations. Another is recognition of the time-intensive nature of a partnership building process. There are many issues related to communications, cultural sensitivity and trust that must be overcome. Thought should be given to these issues in project design.

While it was agreed that there exists gaps in information to determine a direct causal relationship between environmental pollution and health effects, it was also the consensus that the inability to show a direct causal relationship should not hinder prevention and intervention activities. Barriers to determining direct causal relationships include the absence of human exposure and health surveillance information. Another is the lack of health data to better elucidate socioeconomic and racial factors. Lastly, analysis of health impacts "one chemical at a time" precludes an understanding of cumulative environmental and human health effects.

Socioeconomic and cultural factors are important in addressing community health concerns. It was the general consensus that ample evidence exists of a relationship between socioeconomic and/or cultural factors and health effects. This raised the question of the type of scientific disciplines needed to fully understand the cumulative effects of environmental impacts on minority, low-income, and/or indigenous populations. Input should be obtained from social scientists as well as physical scientists.

Interestingly, the majority of the comments and views presented in the report parallel the recommendations contained in the 1994 Federal Interagency Symposium on Health Research and Needs to Ensure Environmental Justice and the 1999 Institute of Medicine Report entitled, *Towards Environmental Justice: Research, Education, and Health Policy Needs*. This suggests that most people have similar concerns and recognize similar gaps in current strategies and activities. The majority of the stakeholders look forward to the discussions at the upcoming NEJAC meeting. They also expressed considerable excitement at the possibilities for stronger partnering and collaboration efforts.

Purpose of the National Environmental Justice Advisory Council (NEJAC) Meeting

The charter of the NEJAC directs that entity to provide independent advice to the Environmental Protection Agency's (EPA) Administrator on areas which may include, the direction, criteria, scope, and adequacy of the EPA's scientific research and demonstration projects, relating to environmental justice. To that end, EPA's Office of Environmental Justice (OEJ) has requested the NEJAC hold an issue-oriented, focused public meeting in Atlanta, Georgia. That meeting will be held May 23nd through 26th, 2000.

The NEJAC meeting will focus on federal efforts to secure disease prevention and health improvement in communities where health disparities exist that may result from, or be exacerbated by, disproportionate effects of environmental pollutants and certain socioeconomic and cultural factors. The meeting will center around three important questions, provided below.

(1) What strategies and areas of research (research in this context encompasses a broad range of studies that may include basic science, applied research, and data collection. These may be carried out by the following: federal, state, tribal or local governments; universities; communities; industry; and/or individuals) should be pursued to achieve more effective, integrated community-based health assessment, intervention, and prevention efforts?

(2) How should these strategies be developed, implemented and evaluated so as to insure substantial participation, integration and collaboration among federal agencies, in partnership with the following: impacted communities; public health, medical and environmental professionals; academic institutions; state, tribal and local governments; and the private sector?

(3) How can consideration of socioeconomic vulnerabilities: a) contribute to a better understanding of health disparities and cumulative and disproportionate environmental effects; and b) be incorporated into community health assessments?

Purpose of the Stakeholder Representatives Interview

In order to have an intensive, focused meeting, the OEJ determined that conducting preliminary interviews of stakeholders would lead to the elucidation of particular issues, which would then serve as the starting point for discussions at the NEJAC meeting. To that end, a number of individuals, representatives from academia; industry/business; federal, state and local governments; community groups; and tribal entities were interviewed. Specific questions were designed by OEJ, with input from the reporter, Dr. Adrienne Hollis. During the summary of the questionnaires, a number of recurring issues and recommendations emerged. Those have been categorized into themes, for use in focusing the NEJAC meeting.

Description of Stakeholder Interviewees

Twenty-one interviews were conducted with stakeholders representing the federal government (6), state health and environmental agencies (3), academic institutions (8), and community organizations (3). In addition, there was one representative from industry/business. These individuals have been involved in some form of community-based activity, including funding research projects, conducting assessment, intervention, evaluation, and/or prevention activities with communities, or by working directly in and with communities. They each bring a wealth of knowledge and expertise to this process. A list of the stakeholders interviewed is provided in Appendix A, and the list of questions utilized during the interview process is provided in Appendix B.

In addition, a draft copy of the initial results of the questionnaire was shared with members of the May 2000 NEJAC Meeting Planning Committee. Their comments and recommendations are also incorporated into this document.

Themes and Accompanying Comments

(1) Developing Effective Partnerships

Who Should Partner in a Community-Based Health Research Model?
There was almost unanimous agreement on the part of stakeholders that the community, or community-based organization was the most critical component for a successful partnership. One community stakeholder, who suggested that academia and community partnerships were the most critical, explained that *"...communities alone will not have the credibility or capacity to address health issues in a way that would lead to policy change, but these partnerships can help communities push a public health agenda...."* They further stated that *"...until the funding process changes, the research needed to do work in communities needs to go through academic institutions...."* A number of stakeholders discussed the definition of 'community'. Some non-community stakeholders pointed out that there should be a mechanism to define community. One stakeholder from a state health/environmental office stated that the community should include *"...people from affected community and folks who are not necessarily affected by an event...pollutants do not know barriers, and may eventually affect other areas..."*. A representative from academia stated that *"...we are also community organizations, we employ from and live in the community...academicians are part of the community...."* A stakeholder from the federal government stated that *"...leadership in communities must be defined by communities...we should not try to define community leadership, let them (the community) identify leaders...."* Other entities that were identified by the majority of the stakeholder representatives as a necessary component included; academic research institutions, federal, state, and local government, health care providers, local environmental and health departments, and funding agencies.

A few representatives (one each from academia and a state health/environmental office, and two from government) felt that industry/business should be included in the partnership, in order to achieve success. Interestingly, one stakeholder from academia was very vocal **against** bringing industry to the partnership. This particular stakeholder stated *"...industry has always done something with an ill intent. They are not to be trusted, and most people are not convinced that they [industry] have the interest of the people at heart...."* In contrast, a stakeholder from the state health/environmental agency stated that *"...industry plays a key role as a stakeholder in this process...industry is not explicitly included in the process...they should not be considered a barrier, but they should be included in the partnership...."*

Critical Elements for Success
When asked what elements were needed for a successful partnership, it was the general opinion of the stakeholders that trust and credibility MUST be established among the partners. As one stakeholder explained *"...trust from the community and from the stakeholders is one of the critical elements for success...."* A second stakeholder from academia stated that *"...partnerships will work if accountability and structure are incorporated into the process...."* The overwhelming majority of the stakeholders agreed that establishing trust and credibility is time and resource intensive, and that this should be recognized and acknowledged by all stakeholders. According to one federal stakeholder, *"...trust is a critical element in any partnership...if you outline what you are going to do, do what you say will do and say what you cannot do, that will go a long way toward establishing trust and credibility...."*

A stakeholder from academia stated that the foundation for this model would be developed with education, training or outreach to the community, to ensure that everyone is *"...on the same page...."*

A second stakeholder from academia stated that *"...It is incumbent upon funding agencies to verify partnerships, to insure that it is not some inequitable, patched together, kind of network. This effort requires the evaluation of whether a partnership described on paper, on a grant application, actually exists and will survive post-funding...."*

(2) Intervention and Prevention Activities

When Should Intervention and Prevention Activities Occur?
Intervention and prevention, two of the components of a community-based health model, generated a great deal of discussion. One federal stakeholder suggested that after assessment is complete, the partners should analyze whether intervention is needed. The partners should first discuss what is meant by intervention, then decide what is needed.

A stakeholder from the community and a representative from the NEJAC May 2000 Planning Committee, both discussed the importance of the "Precautionary Principle", which involves taking appropriate measures to protect public health. Although other stakeholders did not use the term "precautionary principle" in their discussions, most, if not all, felt that in the presence of or threat of adverse health effects, there was no need to wait before initiating intervention/prevention activities. These activities should be a major element of the way business is conducted when dealing with environmental issues. One community stakeholder stated that both intervention and prevention activities must be conducted with the community, not on the community in order to be successful. They further stated that the community believes that any research conducted must include an intervention component. In addition, when dealing with federal agencies in these activities, there should be some protocol or guideline on interaction with the community. For example, when ATSDR conducts public health assessments and health consultations, and when EPA conducts risk assessments, there should be a methodology in place for working with communities.

According to a number of stakeholders, prevention is often placed last, both in design and in thinking, when addressing environmental issues. As one federal stakeholder stated, *"...Individuals who are adept at prevention activities have been trained to look upon it as a 'final step' in the process...."* That stakeholder provide the example of EPA's role in public health, which is for the most part, according to the stakeholder, not health related. Their strongest work is in the area of prevention, looking at enforcement of environmental guidelines and laws. Along those same lines, the National Institute for Environmental Health Sciences (NIEHS) has been attempting to address the prevention portion of the model (along with assessment), and has recently begun looking at prevention efforts.

A number of stakeholders felt that intervention was an area needs more attention. An example provided by a state stakeholder, is the issue of asthma. There is a lack of activity in addressing the incidence of asthma, particularly in children. A second example involves lead exposure and toxicity. A number of stakeholders suggest that appropriate intervention and prevention efforts have not been applied to this issue. In addition, it was suggested that intervention and prevention may not be that different. After a partnership has assessed a problem, they should analyze whether intervention is needed, and then decide on an appropriate intervention.

Barriers to Effective Intervention and Prevention
According to input from a number of members of the NEJAC May 2000 Planning Committee, a major barrier to effective intervention and prevention activities stems from the perception that city, state, county, tribal agencies, and/or municipalities are supportive of the activities of the polluting industry or business. This is true even when dealing with federal facilities. Their interest may be

directed more towards economic interests than the health of the community. According to the Committee members, pollution prevention and enforcement activities should be a major emphasis of these entities when dealing with industry/business.

One stakeholder from a state environmental health office stated that a major barrier is the lack of action on the part of the EPA. He discussed the issue of lead contamination in communities as a major example. He felt that this was an established issue that has had virtually no intervention. He further stated that in order for intervention and prevention activities to work, the federal government could not go directly to communities, the state and local health and environmental regulator entities must be involved.

(3) Community-Based Research

What is Community-Based Research?
Initial discussion surrounded the definition of community-based research. The consensus is that the model has to be **participatory**, with the community as an equal partner, in order to be community-based. It was suggested by a member of the NEJAC May 2000 Planning Committee that the name be changed to "community-based participatory research," to differentiate it from research done "in or to" a community. According to a number of stakeholders, in this model (participatory research), the community has a leadership role in activities planned by the partnership. This is an issue that both NIEHS, through its environmental justice partnership grants, and ATSDR, through the Minority Health Association Foundation grants, have been attempting to address.

Most stakeholders (with the majority from academia and the federal government) stated that research in the community-based health research model should be more broadly designed. The definition of this research should be qualitative, rather than quantitative. Assessment of this model has to be rigorous and detailed, and must include what may be non-conventional methodology, including the use of biomarkers. When discussing risk assessment, EPA must be open to incorporating unconventional data into that model. The design of the model should be done by the partnership with all stakeholder.

A representative from the NEJAC May 2000 Planning Committee stated that it was important to note that there are other types of research, besides participatory, which should not be overlooked, because of the value of the data obtained. No additional details, however, were provided.

In addition, a community representative on the NEJAC May 2000 Planning Committee suggested that there should be some protocol or guideline developed which would allow the community to participate in "agency" research, with the term 'agency' inclusive of academic institutions and other entities conducting research. A stakeholder from academia suggested that efforts be made to promote opportunities to increase technical proficiency or empower local communities to conduct small scale studies, using valid methodologies, such as accepted analytical methods for environmental sampling. Funds should be provided which would allow communities to work with researchers who can train and bring communities 'up to speed' on sampling and research methods. Competition for funding between community organizations, academic institutions, and other organizations to work with a specific community, should be eliminated.

Quality and Quantity of Data Produced
The general consensus of the majority of the stakeholders was that data obtained through community-based efforts are useful. The concern is that because of the size of the population, there may not be

statistical significance, which is a concern when using data to generate policy. One stakeholder from academia stated that there is tension between the desire for rigorous study design and the reality of actually conducting that research in the community. According to another stakeholder, a great deal of data are produced, but there is concern about the internal validity of the design.

One stakeholder suggested that efforts should be made to increase technical proficiency or empower local communities to do small scale studies, using valid methodologies and accepted analytical methods for environmental sampling. This should improve the quality of any data produced.

Data Gaps in Community-Based Efforts
One stakeholder from academia stated that data should be gathered on different levels. For example, data is needed on issues surrounding residential and occupational segregation, racial and economic segregation, gender, schedules of exposure, and links between exposure to hazardous substances in hospitals, to name a few.

In addition to the stakeholders mentioned previously, scientists from the social sciences (sociology, psychology, behavioral sciences, anthropology, psychometrics, etc.) should be included in research activities. The community model would benefit from social science. They have a great deal to offer in the area of social behavior, psychological stress etc.

When dealing with the issue of research, there needs to be some guidelines on how rigorous the research and science needs to be in order to be relevant to policy development. While it is agreed that there should not be tradeoffs between scientific rigor and policy relevance, there needs to be consideration for the value of this type of research. While the data may not meet the certain standards required for scientific rigor, the data can be important in its own right. The question becomes: 'How much research is needed before actions are taken, particularly around issues of health disparities?'

Assessment, Intervention, and Prevention in the Community-Based Research Model
Although all stakeholders agreed with the inclusion of these components in a community-based model, a few stakeholders have suggested that communities have had enough "assessment." Those stakeholders, representatives of community, academia and state health/environmental entities, stated that we are very good at assessment, but need to focus on intervention and prevention activities. In contrast, one federal stakeholder stated that assessment was the element most in need of improvement. It was almost unanimous that communities play a major role in assessment, intervention and prevention. In addition, one federal stakeholder stated that *"...the assessment describes what is or what exists, and what has been done concerning particular issues. ..."* One stakeholder from academia stated that assessment is core, in terms of what kind of data is required. Assessment is also important because community and scientists' perceptions needed to be discussed.

Evaluation in Community-Based Research
A fourth component, in addition to assessment, intervention and prevention, has been suggested by a number of stakeholders, including representatives from the federal government, academia, state health/environmental agencies, and community groups. According to these stakeholders, evaluation should be a major part of any health model. One stakeholder from academia also pointed out that evaluation is also a barrier to implementation of the model, as very few stakeholders are trained to conduct evaluation. Rigorous evaluation is needed throughout the research project, to prevent delayed intervention in some communities. One stakeholder stated that, in the past, evaluation had been conducted via a traditional approach, which does not recognize social assets (i.e., how we build

models or pilot projects that leave the community more empowered). This would require quantitative evaluation. The type of evaluation needed is foreign to researchers, because it *is* qualitative and formative in nature. One stakeholder stated that all partners must feel comfortable with the tools of evaluation, and that training in evaluation should be required for everyone, including the funding agency. A number of stakeholders discussed the need for input from individuals in the social and behavioral sciences, as they would have expertise in evaluation.

One federal stakeholder opined that evaluation is different from assessment. Evaluation is inherent with value, assessment describes what is or what exists concerning particular issues, as well as what has been done. It was also suggested that in addition to the evaluation conducted by the partners, outside evaluation would provide invaluable insight and feedback on the activities conducted.

A community stakeholder stated *"...when people think about evaluation, it is intimidating. We should embrace it. It is usually one way, from the funding agency...it needs to come back the other way - what is the agency internally doing to evaluate how it does its work...."*

(4) Current Models of Community-Based Research

General Comments
The prevalent opinion among stakeholders interviewed, including those from the scientific community, is that there are successful models of community-based research. Several interviewees took note of the following community-based research models. It is beyond the scope of an interview process to describe each in sufficient detail and accuracy. Most suggested that someone should compile the results of those activities, detailing the types of community interactions and the models used. A description of some of these projects can be found in Appendix C.

The majority of these examples incorporate environmental justice principles into the partnership activities, but this is not true for all examples. A general suggestion, made by a stakeholder representative from federal government was to examine the results of grants funded in the past. These grant programs include Environmental Justice Community University Partnerships for Communications (NIEHS), Community-Based Intervention/Prevention Strategies (NIEHS), Environmental Justice Pollution Prevention Grants (EPA), Environmental Justice Community-University Partnerships (EPA), and the Environmental Justice Small Grants (EPA).

It should also be noted that there was general consensus that an evaluation of models currently in use would provide valuable information, as well as provide a number of tools which can be adapted for specific projects.

Critical Elements for Success of the Model
Critical elements for success, as identified by the majority of the stakeholders, include respect, equity and empowerment. According to one stakeholder, *"...respect deals with the fact that culture and community concerns deserve equal merit from the partners. Equity involves sharing the wealth with the community, and empowerment involves being committed to the principle of making the community self sufficient...."*

A number of stakeholders also identified 'having an open mind', and 'stepping outside of the box' is also critical to the success of the project. According to the stakeholders, this involves a willingness to conduct activities differently, to see value in collaboration with other partners. An additional element identified as important to the success of the model, is capacity within each component to work together.

One government stakeholder stated that current risk assessment methodologies are not designed to address non-chemical stressors. They (risk assessments) are not epidemiological studies. Consideration should be taken in addressing this issue.

Barriers to the Success of the Model
Special attention should be given to specific identifiable barriers to the success of the model. One such barrier, identified by state health/environment, community, and academic stakeholders, is the lack of capacity-building for community based organizations, to enable them to partner with scientists and health care providers. A second barrier is the time intensive activities needed in the initial stages of the partnership development. The consensus among the stakeholders that the time-intensive nature of the partnership could be a barrier, from a funding perspective as well as a commitment (by stakeholders) perspective. An additional barrier is the complexity of the model design. The more complex the model, the more difficult it is to plan, implement and evaluate. This is true for any model. Other barriers identified by numerous stakeholders included resources, such as computer equipment, and economic issues (including simple issues such as travel of community members to partnership meetings).

One stakeholder from academia discussed institutional barriers, related to tribal council changes and cultural sensitivities as a major impediment to the success of the model.

A community member stated that the barriers around relationship are not as important when community capacity is built-in. The focus becomes more on prevention and dealing with the current exposure than trying to figure out what happened in the past.

(5) Barriers and Data Gaps and their Relationship to Health Effects

While it is agreed that there are a number of barriers and data gaps in current research activities directed toward addressing health effects, it is also the consensus of the majority of the stakeholders that the inability to show a causal relationship between exposure and effect should not hinder prevention and intervention activities. One of the barriers identified time and again, is the continual effort to determine past exposure and health effect. It has been suggested that efforts should focus on dealing with current exposure instead.

One federal stakeholder stated that the work started in the 1985 Secretary's Task Force on Black and Minority Health Report, which identified both the current state of the health of people of color and the data gaps, is the place to start. That stakeholder also stated that the Institute of Medicine Report on Environmental Justice would prove invaluable. Other resources mentioned include the National Medical Association, the Hispanic Health Association, and organizations for Asian and Native Americans.

When asked what the three greatest barriers to determining the relationship between exposure and health effects, one federal stakeholder stated that little is known about the latency period between exposure and health effect. There is also the perception that health and environment are not related. The environment has not been associated with adverse health effects in the past. A number of stakeholders from academia stated that the type of exposure is important, and that it is difficult to determine, given the latency period, what the exposure was.

Another barrier identified is the issue of an absence of sufficient human exposure and health surveillance information, beyond that provided through the Toxic Release Inventory (TRI) or emissions data. In addition, although health data is collected by race and ethnicity, there are no indicators of social class on the birth certificate, no information on income, health insurance, etc. This makes it difficult to determine the impact of race versus socioeconomic status when examining health effects. One federal stakeholder identified the definition of 'health' as a barrier. He stated that health is not an outcome, it is a process which leads to an outcome. That outcome must be defined by an individual group.

One community stakeholder stated that one barrier is the procedure used which only analyzes one chemical at a time, instead of studying synergistic effects. In addition, they stated that little information is available on new chemicals, and transient exposures (the effects of exposure at different times in our life...past and current exposure). An additional barrier mentioned is poor health record keeping, where people receive services from different clinics, with no uniform way to keep track. In addition, the lack of a universal health plan was identified by the community stakeholder as a barrier.

(6) Socioeconomic Vulnerabilities and Cultural Factors

The overwhelming consensus is that all socioeconomic and cultural factors are important in addressing community health concerns. According to one stakeholder, risk factors are socioeconomic and behavioral, so interventions must be the same. These factors include social, behavioral, economic, cultural, and political issues. It is the general consensus of stakeholders that ample evidence exists of a relationship between socioeconomic and /or cultural factors and health impacts. A federal stakeholder stated that "*...you cannot assume that issues around race and ethnicity are the same as those surrounding socioeconomic concerns...holding demographics constant, race and ethnicity continue to be significant, holding race constant, demographics and ethnicity are significant and so on....*"

According to one academician, socioeconomic conditions and health, absolute and relative poverty, standard of living, access to healthy foods, position at work (occupational environment), are all factors relevant to health. They continued by stating that "*...culture includes behavioral differences, cultural disparities, such as language barriers, culture mixed with racism, etc.,.....*"

Interviewees recognized socioeconomic vulnerabilities and cultural factors as being important contributors to health disparities. Consideration and attention need to be directed at the role of other factors, such as psychological stressors (i.e., job security, safety issues, housing, etc.), class, outside stressors, environmental stressors, economic and racial segregation and others, may play in relation to health disparities.

One stakeholder from academia stated "*...if you are talking about environmental justice, you must discuss issues of class in relation to race, gender, and other factors. This should include informed social scientist' input, not just physical science...*"

(7) Effective Risk Communication

It was the general opinion of most stakeholders that in order for a partnership to be successful and for community-based research to be effective, all stakeholders should be able to communicate with each other. One federal stakeholder stated that "*...we have to find a way to talk to communities about what* *we can and cannot do in a better way. This should be different from the risk assessor coming in and calculating risk, or saying that they cannot calculate it...scientists and policy makers have to be more helpful to communities, or they will lose credibility....*" According to one federal stakeholder, "*...the key is communication, we do not talk each other's language (i.e., toxicology, chemistry, etc., tend to resolve problems, but need to learn to listen better...they fail the community as scientists....*" A number of stakeholders stated that communication was especially important when a representative from the medical profession is speaking with lay people about health issues or an academician is speaking about research in scientific terms, or when a risk assessor or health assessor is speaking in technical terms.

Quite a number of stakeholder representatives stated that, in order to avoid confusion and misunderstandings later in the partnership, expectations and limitations of *EACH* entity should be identified in the initial stages of development. As one stakeholder stated "*...communication, good up-front understanding of the capabilities and limitations are essential....*" In addition, the community's (or any other stakeholders') perception of risk should be taken into account when determining or communicating risk.

A stakeholder from academia suggested that all partners receive some training in effective risk communication before activities are initiated. In addition, cultural competency is important when attempting a risk communication effort. An example of this was presented by a federal stakeholder. In efforts to address pollution at the United States and Mexican border, a number of documents were developed, for different educational levels. This major risk communication effort was very successful. According to that same stakeholder, the goal of risk communication is understanding, not consensus. A second stakeholder from academia stated that we need to be conscious of how risk is communicated. The meetings where information is provided should be continuous consensus building sessions. There needs to be growth and updating of activities occurring since the last meeting. The connection and partnership should be one in which the lines of communication should have already been open, there should be no surprises.

All stakeholders must agree, as a part of their initial standards of conduct, to accept the information provided, even though it may not be the particular results/conclusions they were expecting. If trust and credibility have been established, this will occur as a normal part of the partnership interactions.

(8) Sustainability

Sustainability of the Community-based Health Model
This particular topic, sustainability, is related to a number of issues. Most stakeholders identified the need for the community-based health model must be sustainable. It must contain certain strategies for building capacity, so that activities continue, even after the funding period ends. To that end, resources are an integral part of sustainability. Both sustainability of the partnership (the model) and of the planned intervention were identified as resource intensive activities.

Sustainability of the Activities
As mentioned earlier, the initial activities, where trust and credibility are established, are time intensive. Most stakeholders, the majority from academia, believe that funding entities must take into consideration the fact that this effort will be time and resource intensive, particularly when placing time limits on grants. For example, a one year funding period is not feasible for establishing a partnership and initiating activities. Funds should be set aside to create partnerships for projects that

are beneficial to everyone, that do not cost billions of dollars, and that will allow stakeholders (academia, community, etc.) to work together, instead of competing for limited funds.

As one NEJAC May 2000 Planning Committee member stated, there should be some way to determine, other than the ending of the funding period, when it is time to end a project. In some cases, if the research goes further than the allotted time, it will impact agencies and entities that were thought to be out of reach. This type of success would only be due to the sustained efforts of the partners involved.

(9) Federal Agencies as Partners

Role of Federal Agencies in Partnerships
Most stakeholders stated that before federal agencies can partner with communities and other organizations, they must first learn to work together. Currently, the prevailing thought among stakeholders is that federal agencies are each "doing their own thing", addressing their agenda, although there are some agencies that are attempting to establish a more coordinated working relationship with others. For example, the National Institutes of Health is trying to create a cross-initiative around health disparities.

A number of federal agencies were identified as potential partners in a community based model. Most stakeholders agree that the appropriate federal agencies would simply depend on the issue(s) which need to be addressed through the model. Some agencies identified include EPA, ATSDR, CDC, DHHS, DOE, USDA, FDA, OSHA, DOT, HUD. Other agencies should be willing and waiting to participate, as the need arises and they are identified by the partnership.

Also, as partners in this process, federal agencies should realize the time it takes to form partnerships, and be willing to provide funds to conduct appropriate activities.

The Role of Federal Agencies in Addressing Health Disparities
According to one academician, the current problem federal agencies face when addressing health disparities stems from the idea that their role is stove-piped. For example, one agency may be studying asthma, another may be concentrating on genetics, while a third may be focused on surveillance. He further stated that these agencies have tunnel vision, and should attempt to develop an integrated plan to attack health disparities. They should also move toward a more integrated effort for exposure data gathering. A second stakeholder from academia stated that they have been encouraged by the explosion of interest of federal agencies in addressing health disparities. The level of interest and willingness to fund projects by NIEHS, the National Institute on Aging, the National Cancer Institute, CDC and others has been good.

One federal stakeholder opined that a second role of federal agencies is assurance and policy development, as outlined in the IOM report. The policy development is at the federal, state, and local level. A second stakeholder stated that state and federal government are involved in monitoring health, and that a good contact person for information on this effort would be Dr. Diane Rowley from the CDC.

OTHER STAKEHOLDER COMMENTS

Some important stakeholder comments were not included in the main part of the document, as they did not lend themselves to any particular theme. They are nonetheless, important. Those comments are provided here.

One comment from a federal stakeholder was "…we know what to do, we don't have the courage to do it. It is not an issue of health, but an issue of liability. Whose responsibility is it? That is a whole set of issues that do not get resolved. This is an overwhelming issue. There are so many unanswered questions…when in doubt, we should err on the side of public health. We don't have to wait for illness or risk factors before doing something. That is almost unethical. Why wait for the dead bodies...."

A representative from academia stated that "...*it is wonderful that attention is being paid to the importance of developing community based models. This activity needs real resources, lip service and not following through will cause more problems and distress...*"

A comment that was made by a stakeholder from the community and academia, is that a mechanism be provided to educate youth so that they may continue the work started by these individuals.

APPENDIX A

ENVIRONMENTAL JUSTICE STAKEHOLDER INTERVIEWEE LIST

STAKEHOLDER INTERVIEWEE LIST

1. Mr. Michael Callahan — EPA Office of Research and Development
2. Dr. David Carpenter — School of Public Health, University of Albany, SUNY
3. Mr. Cecil Corbin Mark — WHEACT
4. Ms. Carolyn Covey-Morris — SOCMA, VP Government Relations and Public Affairs (Industry/Business)
5. Dr. Allen Dearry — National Institute of Environmental Health Sciences
6. Ms. Paula Goode — EPA Office of Children's Health
7. Dr. Richard Gragg — Environmental Sciences Institute, Florida A&M University
8. Dr. Walter Handy — Cincinnati Health Department
9. Dr. Cynthia Harris — Institute of Public Health, Florida A&M University
10. Dr. Bruce Kennedy — Health and Social Behavior, Harvard University School
11. Dr. Patrick Kinney — Columbia University School of Public Health
12. Dr. Nancy Krieger — Harvard School of Public Health
13. Dr. Paula Lantz — University of Michigan
14. Ms. Yin Ling Leung — Asian Reproduction Rights
15. Dr. Andrew McBride — North Carolina Department of Health
16. Dr. Karen Medville — Arizona State University, West. American Indian Environmental Health Sciences Program
17. Dr. Ngozi Oleru — Environmental Health Department, Seattle Health Department
18. Dr. Bill Sanders — EPA OPPT/OPPTS
19. Ms. Samara Swanston — The Watch Person Project
20. Dr. Reuben Warren — The Agency for Toxic Substances and Disease Registry

21. Dr. Hal Zenick   EPA's Office of Research and Development

OTHER PLANNED INTERVIEWEES

22. Ms. Katsi Cook   Akwasasne Nation (could not be interviewed due to scheduling conflicts)

23. Mr. Michael Sage   National Center for Environmental Health, Centers for Disease Control and Prevention (could not be interviewed due to scheduling conflicts)

24. Another Industry Representative   Several unsuccessful attempts were made to find an additional industry representative.

APPENDIX B

CONVENER'S QUESTIONS FOR STAKEHOLDER REPRESENTATIVES

CONVENER'S QUESTIONS

The EPA seeks advice and recommendations from the National Environmental Justice Advisory Council (NEJAC) on Federal efforts to improve the health status of communities. In particular, EPA asks the NEJAC to focus on communities where health disparities exist and in which those disparities are associated with: environmental stressors; and certain socioeconomic and/or cultural factors.

(1) Community-Based Public Health Model

The Agency is considering how programs/projects/activities that will address community-based health concerns can be designed and implemented with the direct involvement of all stakeholders (community, industry, local government/tribal entities, academic institutions, and State and Federal agencies). It has been suggested that this integrated, community-based model should include three components: assessment, intervention, and prevention. In the questions below, the phrase "community-based health model," includes these three components and substantial stakeholder involvement.

(1) Do you think that this model is a viable one for addressing community health concerns?

(b) Are there barriers to implementation of this community-based health model, in general, and with your agency or organization or community, including tribal groups, in particular?

(2) Design, Implementation and Evaluation of the Community-Based Health Model

(1) How should each of the components (e.g., assessment, intervention, and prevention) of this community-based health model be designed, implemented, and evaluated?

(2) Who should design, implement, and evaluate each or all of these components?

(3) What research would be most useful in the area of community-based health design, implementation, and evaluation (e.g., methodology, data, etc.)?

(3) Examples of Community-Based Health Efforts in Action/Practice
(1) Can you give an example of a community-based health model in action/practice and how it was conducted?

(2) What methodology did it follow?

(3) Was this program successful, and, if so, why?

(4) What was the result(s) of these efforts?
(i) Did significant actions result (e.g., abatement, new policies, or research) or changes in stakeholder relationships?
(ii) Which stakeholders were involved in affecting these actions?
(iii) What did each stakeholder bring to the process?

(iv) Would increased involvement by any particular stakeholder group have made the effort more successful?

(4) Critical Elements for Success

    (1) What specific elements (e.g., policies, activities, and methodologies/approaches) of each component are required for the success of this community-based health model?

    (2) For each component, which elements are most in need of improvement?

    (3) What specific research would help bring about these improvements?

(5) Environmental Justice

    (1) Were environmental justice concerns incorporated into the actions described above?

    (2) How in particular where these concerns integrated and/or addressed?

(6) Partnerships

    (1) Which partnerships are most critical to the success of a community-based health model, and why?

    (2) Are you aware of examples of successful partnerships among stakeholders, including appropriate Federal agencies? Why were these partnerships successful?

    (3) Which Federal Agencies should partner in community-based health efforts, and in which specific component(s)?

    (4) What can be done to promote the formation and use of partnerships among stakeholders, in general?

    (5) What research would be most useful in this area?

(7) Federal Agency's Role

    (1) What is the current role of Federal agencies in addressing health disparities in communities?

    (2) What should be the role of Federal agencies in addressing health disparities in communities?

(8) Quality and Quantity of Data Produced Through Community-Based Efforts

- (1) Are data produced through community-based health assessments/research useable when drawing conclusions, testing hypotheses, and/or making policy recommendations?

- (2) What types of data gaps are most frequently associated with community-based efforts?

- (3) What research would be most useful to address data gaps?

(9) Consideration of Socioeconomic and/or Cultural Factors in Addressing Community Health Concerns through Assessment, Intervention, and Prevention

- (1) Are specific socioeconomic and/or cultural factors relevant to addressing community health concerns? Which ones?

- (2) Is there a scientific basis or relationship between socioeconomic and/or cultural factors and health impacts? If so, which ones?

- (3) What research would be most useful in addressing these issues?

(10) Relationship Between Exposure and Health Effect

- (1) What are the three greatest barriers to determining the relationship between exposure and health effects?

- (2) What role have community-based efforts played in resolving issues of exposure and health effect? Can you provide examples?

- (3) What areas of research or data collection would be most useful in these areas?

(11) What other suggestions would you like to make?

APPENDIX C

Models of Community-Based Research

THE AKWESASNE FIRST ENVIRONMENT RESTORATION INITIATIVE (Principal Investigator: Mary Arquette)

OBJECTIVES:
- Develop partnerships among community members, health care providers, and research scientists.

- Design community-based strategies for environmental health education, outreach, and training in the Akwesasne Mohawk community, which is adjacent to a Superfund site with a history of major environmental contamination.

METHODS:
- An initial needs assessment examining health risks, perception of risks, and communication of risks will be conducted using focus groups.
- Develop educational materials with Mohawk language content and symbolism.
- Produce an air of "Good Health" show on Akwesasne Mohawk Radio.
- Conduct environmental health fairs at local schools.
- Implement training workshops for clinicians and traditional practitioners wit a focus on toxic exposures.
- Establish focus groups and workshops to ensure community input into health research needs.

LOCATION:
The Mohawk Nation at Akwesasne (ST. Regis Mohawk Tribe), located in the Great Lakes Basin-St. Lawrence River watershed, is exposed to hazards resulting from the rapid transition from an agricultural to an industrial environment. PCBs have been found in fish, which provide a protein staple in the Mohawk diet and in human breast milk.

DINE COLLEGE - URANIUM EDUCATION IN THE NAVAJO NATION (Principal Investigator: Mark C. Bauer)

OBJECTIVES:
- Establish collaboration among the Navajo community, Navajo Community College, local primary care physicians, the Centra0 Consolidated School District, the University of New Mexico Center for Health Promotion for Rural American Indians, and scientists with expertise in radiation health issues.
- Conduct qualitative and quantitative research with the Navajo community concerning knowledge and behavior about radiation.
- Produce culturally appropriate educational materials about cancer, birth defects, and radiation.
- Conduct community programs and training sessions leading to greater awareness regarding radiation dangers.

METHODS:
- Establish a radiation education center for the Navajos in geographic areas affected by uranium mining.
- Assess community-identified concerns, priorities, values, goals, and strategies for education on radiation issues.
- Develop culturally appropriate education and communication materials based on the preliminary community assessment.
- Provide in-depth training of community leaders and health care providers.
- Develop and implement education, training, and organizing strategies for grassroots community members.
- Perform community-based evaluation of project's effectiveness to determine its progress in attaining community-defining goals.

LOCATIONS:

- The Navajo Nation in NM, AZ, and UT contains >225,000 people, only half of whom have graduated from high school. Uranium mines operated from 1940 - 1980. Radioactive uranium tailings were freely dumped. Lung cancer, silicosis, renal toxicity, and other disorders occur at a high rate.

ASIAN AND PACIFIC ISLANDERS FOR PRODUCTIVE HEALTH (Principal Investigator: Yin L. Leung)

OBJECTIVES:
- Create a core group of Southeast Asian girl leaders that are knowledgeable and skilled in educating other community people about environmental hazards and reproductive health.
- Improve reproductive health services through joint work with family planning clinics that serve these communities.
- Build capacity between two project sites so communities will recognize their common environmental justice and reproductive problems.
- Seeks to redress the environmental impact Southeast Asians experienced because of the Vietnam War, to eliminate current exposures issues today and to improve communities reproductive and overall health and well-being.

METHODS:
- Recruit and train a core of Southeast Asians girls on basic issues of environmental justice and reproductive health to become community trainers.
- Use participatory action research, a systematic investigation with the collaboration of those affected by the issue being studied, fro purposes of education and taking action or affecting social change, to improve the health and environment of these communities.

LOCATIONS:
- Long Beach, California
- Richmond and Oakland, California
  Following the Vietnam War, refugees from Southeast Asia settled in the United States. Exposed to numerous chemicals during the war, they arrived with little money and no job or language skills, settling in poor and environmentally hazardous areas. Due to lack of education and jobs skills they work primarily in menial jobs putting them at additional risk of exposure both at work and at home.

URBAN APPALACHIAN COUNCIL LOWER PRICE HILL ENVIRONMENTAL LEADERSHIP COALITION (Principal Investigator: Pauletta Hansel)

OBJECTIVES:
- Promote neighborhood leadership that has the information, skills, and resources for successful approaches to environmental pollution, risk communication, and public health service.
- Identify and implement changes to procedures used to address the unique environmental quality and health status problems of historically under served communities affects by environmental pollution.
- Develop a long-term working relationship among residents and community organizations in Lower Price Hill, the University of Cincinnati, and the Cincinnati Health Department.

METHODS:

- Design and conduct a survey of the community regarding health concerns and environment pollution.
- Develop education and training modules to maintain effective communication between the Lower Price Hill Environmental Leadership Coalition and the community.
- Develop evaluation materials to be used to determine effectiveness of the project.

LOCATIONS:
- Lower Price Hill, located in Cincinnati, Ohio, is an urban Appalachian community. Residents are predominantly low-income Caucasians; 71% have not completed high school, compared to 28% for the city, as a whole; unemployment is >20%; 90% of concentrations of lead have been found in playgrounds. Children exhibit learning disabilities at twice the rate of children from other neighborhoods and are five times more likely to suffer from acute respiratory infections.

THE SOUTHERN CALIFORNIA ENVIRONMENTAL HEALTH PROJECT (Principal Investigator: Carlos Porras)

OBJECTIVES:
- Institute a collaboration among community representatives, local health care providers, and university researchers.
- Educate community members and health care providers and promote adoption of pollution prevention measures.
- Establish a community-based strategy for reducing community and worker exposure to environmental pollutants.

METHODS:
- Identify leaders in the targeted community, involving 8 cities, and in the medical community.
- Analyze existing environmental data in the targeted community to identify data gaps.
- Identify priority community health issues through surveys and focus groups.
- Educate residents, workers, and medical providers.
- Develop and implement a pilot program that offers solutions to identified environmental health problems.
- Develop and implement exposure reduction strategies, with an emphasis on pollution prevention measures.

LOCATION:
- South East Los Angeles includes a number of pollution sources, e.g., highly industrialized tracts where chemicals are released, severe urban smog, occupational exposures, and lead poisoning. This zip code area is the dirtiest subregion within the State of California. The area is home to a low-income population, approximately 87% Hispanic/Latino.

RURAL COALITION - THE COMMUNITY-RESPONSIVE PARTNERS FOR ENVIRONMENTAL HEALTH (Principal Investigator: Lorette Picciano-Hanson)

OBJECTIVES:
- Develop a partnership among members of a National Advisory Board of community representatives, local health care providers, and environmental health scientists.

- Implement a partnership model in two communities which will develop specific collaborative projects to achieve measurable results in identifying, preventing, and mitigating exposures.
- Build competency in environmental health assessment and community training.

METHODS:
- Help train the targeted communities to define the problem, analyze the causes, research the solutions, and develop community strategies to solve the problem.
- Train community members to conduct exposure assessment, focusing on development of skills in analysis, record keeping, and attention to detail and protocols.
- Train health care providers in occupational and environmental medicine.
- Empower community to reduce exposure to hazards through education and training.

LOCATIONS:
- Sumter County, AL. Contains the largest toxic waste dump in the U.S. Seventy percent African-American.
- El Paso, TX. Farmworker community in West, TX.

CLARK UNIVERSITY--NUCLEAR RISK MANAGEMENT FOR NATIVE COMMUNITIES (NRMNC) (Principal Investigator: Dianne P. Quigley)

OBJECTIVES:
- Establish collaboration among investigators at Clark University in Worcester, MA and Native American community and health care organizations in Oklahoma and Nevada.
- Increase awareness in Native American communities exposed to radiation contamination from DOE sites.
- Enable these communities to resolve health concerns related to radiation contamination in their environment.

METHODS:
- Identify priority community health research and information needs.
- Develop a "train the trainers" program via collaboration among scientists, community representatives, and health care providers.
- Implement community and health care education modules.
- Design and implement a plan for risk management and prevention activities.
- Share relevant materials and strategies with other Native American communities.

LOCATIONS:
- Western Shoshone Nation near the Nevada Test Site.
- Cherokee Nation at Sequoyah Fuels, OK, a uranium processing facility in operation for 23 years.

LAOTIAN ORGANIZING PROJECT OF THE ASIAN PACIFIC ENVIRONMENTAL NETWORK, RICHMOND LAOTIAN ENVIRONMENTAL JUSTICE COLLABORATION (Principal Investigator: Peggy K. Saika)

OBJECTIVES:
- Develop a model of research, outreach, education, and communication that addresses the immediate environmental health needs of the communities population.
- Build community capacity to understand environmental health issues.

- Develop appropriate tools to reach this limited-English-speaking population.

METHODS:
- Representatives from the main Laotian tribal groups will participate in recruitment and training of community organizers.
- Design needs assessment strategy and implement community outreach and publicity activities.
- Develop a training curriculum for 39 community advocates to carry out the needs assessment.
- Train community advocates on environmental hazards including location of toxic sites relative to where Laotians live and garden, consumption of fish, occupational health and safety issues, and determine understanding of lead hazards and knowledge of available interventions.

LOCATION:
- Richmond, CA. Over 350 industrial facilities encircle Richmond, including waste incinerators, oil refineries, pesticide and fertilizer plants, and other chemical manufacturers. Laotians in the area have the highest percentage of contaminants from urban gardens and fish. Few are English literate.

UNIVERSITY OF MARYLAND SCHOOL OF MEDICINE, BALTIMORE ENVIRONMENTAL JUSTICE YOUTH PROJECT (Principal Investigator: Barbara Sattler)

OBJECTIVES:
- Increase awareness and understanding of urban environmental health issues.
- Organize a city-wide Environmental Justice Youth Conference (EJYC).
- Develop a comprehensive health assessment plan to be used by non-expert community residents.
- Initiate an environmental health awareness program focused on asthma.

METHODS:
- Characterize the distribution of air pollutants and evaluate the contributions of hazardous particles emitted from major sources, including incinerators and diesel emissions.
- Train students in environmental health research via participation in data collection and analysis.
- Introduce students to the complexity of environmental regulatory and policy decisions as they evaluate research results.
- In conjunction with Adolescent Clinics, the EJYC will help develop an awareness program for teens on environmentally related respiratory problems with a focus on asthma.

LOCATION:
- Baltimore, MD. A wide array of environmental insults, including: poor air quality; aging industry with variable environmental controls; older housing stock with lead contamination; diesel powered buses; significant rodent and pest problems; inadequate delivery of basic services. Inner-city Baltimore HS students, mostly African-American, constitute EJYC.

WEST HARLEM ENVIRONMENTAL JUSTICE PARTNERSHIP: EXPANDING THE COMMUNITY RESEARCH AGENDA (Principal Investigator: Peggy M. Shepard)

OBJECTIVES:
- Inform and empower predominantly low income people of color about the disproportionate levels of pollutants to which they are exposed.

- Establish effective communication linkages between community residents, environmental health researchers, and health care providers who live and work in West Harlem.
- Develop environmental health leadership around identified hazards through education and training provided by environmental health researchers and health educators.
- Document and evaluate the efficacy of the proposed project to enhance awareness and understanding of environmental health concerns that impact Northern Manhattan communities.

METHODS:
- Hold public forums at which environmental issues that impact neighborhoods will be addressed.
- Provide training sessions for health care providers on environmental health awareness.
- Recruit, train, and certify twenty residents from each community on environmental health concepts and issues, including environmental justice, Develop leadership training manual and informational pamphlets for use in training sessions and during planned presentations.

LOCATIONS:
- Cental Harlem, population of 115,000, 85% African-American, 10% Latino, 41% unemployed.
- West Harlem, population 107,000, 39% African-American, 36% Latino, 19% Caucasian; 73% new arrivals are from Dominican Republic.
- Washington Heights, population 190,000, 18% African-American, 67% Latino (mostly Dominican), 15% Caucasian. There are a wide variety of outdoor and indoor environmental exposures affecting residents of these areas, including particulate matter and carbon monoxide generated by truck and bus traffic, sulfates and nitrates from a sewage treatment plant, lead paint, and allergenic debris from roaches and rodents.

UNIVERSITY OF MASSACHUSETTS--LOWELL SOUTHEAST ASIAN ENVIRONMENTAL JUSTICE PARTNERSHIP (Principal Investigator: Linda Silka)

OBJECTIVES:
- Increase community awareness of basic environmental health concepts, issues, and resources.
- Ensure the community has an ongoing role in identifying and defining problems and environmental risk.
- Ensure health providers and environmental health scientists are aware of environmental risks and concerns of community residents.

METHODS:
- Develop a working partnership among the Southeast Asian groups in Lowell that will provide a culturally organized focus for identification of environmental health problems with the community.
- Develop a culturally appropriate media presentation, including geographic information systems, to serve as a stimulus to assess environmental health priority concerns as perceived by the community.

- Begin a process of solving identified problems and focus on how to sustain community activism.

LOCATION:
- Lowell, MA contains a Superfund site and 97 additional confirmed and suspected hazardous waste sites. It ranks fourth in the state in rate of reported toxic released and has a long history of industrial contamination. The county is fourth in the nation in hazardous waste generation and ninth in industrial air emission from incinerators. Many of the residents are Southeast Asian, mostly Cambodian and Laotian.

SILICONE VALLEY TOXICS COALITION --SILICONE VALLEY ENVIRONMENTAL HEALTH & JUSTICE PROJECT (Principal Investigator: Theodore G. Smith)

OBJECTIVES:
- Enable low-income minority communities to identify and effectively address toxic chemical hazards where they live, work, and play.
- Improve the health of the community and workers by increasing knowledge of and reducing exposure to hazardous chemicals.
- Promote pollution prevention and improved health and safety practices within the high tech electronics industry and the related service sectors.

METHODS:
- Produce educational materials, conduct educational outreach including cultural programming and conduct a public awareness media campaign.
- Develop and implement a training program for community members and medical care providers.
- Promote institutional change and policy development to reduce and prevent toxic exposures.
- Develop and sustain partnership of community, scientists, and health professionals, recruit members and develop leaders for community-based organizations and develop the organizational capacity and funding to sustain the project over time.

LOCATION:
- Santa Clara County, CA
  The area known as Silicone Valley is home to the electronics industry and contains 29 Superfund sites. A large percentage of the is comprised of people of color, the majority of whom live near the sites and work in the industries that contribute to the contamination.

UNIVERSITY OF NORTH CAROLINA, CHAPEL HILL--SOUTHEAST HALIFAX ENVIRONMENTAL REAWAKENING (Principal Investigator: Stephen B. Wing)

OBJECTIVES:
- Expand environmental health knowledge of Halifax County citizens and health professionals.
- Increase local participation in prevention and remediation of environmental health problems.
- Improve environmental health in the rural South by supporting grassroots leadership and community empowerment.
- Develop education and organizing material for use in other areas; provide outreach to communicate in ten eastern North Carolina counties; offer training in rural environmental health and environmental justice issues to public health students.

METHODS:
- Present collaboratively developing training materials and workshops on environmental health issues to community members.
- Provide quantitative analysis of the racial and socioeconomic characteristics of areas that host intensive livestock operations.

LOCATIONS:
- Tillery, Halifax County, NC
- Counties comprising the Black Belt in Eastern NC.
  Intensive hog operations have rapidly increased in this area over the last decade. NC now ranks second in the country in hog production. Ground water pollution is a particular threat to poor rural residents who depend on shallow wells.

III.D Indigenous Peoples Subcommittee, *Recommendations Concerning the Environmental Health and Research Needs Within Indian Country and Alaska Native Villages*, August 14, 2000

INDIGENOUS PEOPLES SUBCOMMITTEE

OF THE

NATIONAL ENVIRONMENTAL JUSTICE ADVISORY COUNCIL

Recommendations Concerning the Environmental Health and Research Needs
Within Indian Country and Alaska Native Villages

August 14, 2000

BACKGROUND

Indian tribal governments possess a unique political and legal status in the United States. Tribes have long been recognized as separate sovereigns possessing broad inherent authority over their members and territories, however, tribes also are subject to applicable federal law. As governments, the relationship between federally recognized tribes and the federal government is described as "government-to-government" and, in 1994, President Clinton directed each federal agency to operate within this relationship[1] and to maintain it through meaningful consultation and coordination with tribes.[2] Moreover, the federal government owes a special obligation, known as the trust responsibility, toward federally recognized Indian tribes to protect their status as self-governing entities and their property rights. The trust responsibility is based on treaties, statutes, executive orders, and the historical relations between the federal government and tribes. Significantly, it is this trust responsibility that distinguishes federally recognized tribes from all other ethnic and minority groups.

There are some 556 federally recognized tribal governments in the United States, including 223 Alaska Native villages.[3] At the time of the 1990 census, about 1.9 million American Indians/Alaska Natives ("AI/ANs") lived in the United States.[4] In 1993, the Bureau of Indian Affairs estimated that 1.2 million AI/ANs lived within Indian country on lands reserved for their tribes as permanent homelands.[5] "Indian country," which includes reservations, dependent Indian communities, and Indian allotments, comprises approximately 53 million acres of land, much of which is found in remote areas of the nation.[6] The remaining AI/ANs live in urban areas and comprise a growing segment of the Native population.

Commonly cited statistics all seem to agree that AI/AN's economic wealth, public health, and education are the worst of any group in the nation. Poverty and unemployment rates among AI/ANs are the highest for any ethnic group in the country, and education, per capita income, and home ownership are among the lowest.[7] One out of every three AI/ANs lives below the poverty line; approximately 90,000 AI/AN families are homeless or underhoused; and one out of every five AI/AN households lacks adequate plumbing.[8] The statistics are even more disheartening for Alaska Native villages. Only 40% of Alaska Native families have basic sanitation services such as piped drinking water and flush toilets, and more than half of these systems are rudimentary at best.[9] Climate poses a significant challenge to the use of conventional sanitation systems in these communities, which are typically far removed from urban areas. And, the lack of economic development in most Alaska Native villages makes it impossible for these subsistence-based families to pay the cost of bringing in appropriate and sustainable sanitation services.[10]

Health care data on AI/ANs is scarce and unreliable. Significantly, the health status of AI/ANs is far below the health status of the general population in this country, and unmet AI/AN health needs are alarmingly high. This disparity in health status is reflected clearly in the death rates for AI/ANs. For example, AI/ANs have the highest suicide rate (70% higher than the rate for the general population) and the lowest life expectancy of any population in this hemisphere except Haitians.[11] Compared to death rates for all other races in the United States, AI/ANs have a death rate for diabetes mellitus that is 249% higher; a death rate for pneumonia and influenza that is 71% higher; a death rate for tuberculosis that is 533% higher; and a death rate from alcoholism that is 627% higher.[12]

AI/ANs also have a unique set of cancer problems ranging from inadequate screening to under-diagnosis and -reporting of cancer to lack of access to quality health care and new cancer treatments. For example, the leading cause of death for AIs is lung cancer, and AN women have the highest cancer and lung cancer mortality rates of any major racial female group.[13] Recently, the Association of American Indian Physicians reported that cancer is the third leading cause of death for all AI/ANs of all ages; the second leading cause of death for all AI/ANs over age 45; and the leading cause of death for AN women. The Association also reported that, in most parts of the country, AI/ANs have poorer survival rates from cancer than do whites, African Americans, Hispanics, and Asians.[14]

AI/ANs are particularly susceptible to health impacts from pollution due to their traditional and cultural uses of natural resources and, in fact, AI/AN "have greater exposure risks than the general population as a result of their dietary practices and unique cultures that embrace the environment."[15] Fishing, hunting, and gathering often are part of a spiritual, cultural, social, and economic lifestyle, and the survival of many AI/ANs depends on subsistence hunting, fishing, and gathering. In some instances, the right to engage in these activities is legally protected by treaty. Additionally, many AI/ANs also use water, plants, and animals in their traditional and religious practices and ceremonies. As a result, contamination of the water, soil, plants, and animals and the subsequent accumulation of these contaminants in the people through ingestion and contact[16] not only endangers the health of AI/ANs, but also threatens the well-being of their future generations[17] and undermines the cultural survival of tribes and Alaska Native villages.

Significantly, where such traditional, cultural, and subsistence activities are involved, federal and state environmental standards used to protect the general non-Indian/non-Native population may not afford tribes and Alaska Native villages adequate protection from environmental harm.[18] Although several of the major federal environmental laws have been amended to allow federally recognized tribes to assume primacy for certain programs,[19] to date, only a few tribes have Environmental Protection Agency- approved or -promulgated environmental programs.[20] Thus, it is the strong view of the Indigenous Peoples Subcommittee ("IPS") that federally recognized tribes and AI/ANs suffer a disproportionate burden of health consequences due to their exposure to pollutants and hazardous substances in the environment. This is particularly so for AI/AN infants and children.[21]

RECOMMENDATIONS

In developing recommendations for the Environmental Protection Agency on how it can better assess, understand, and address the environmental health research issues and concerns within Indian country and Alaska Native villages, the IPS identified the following questions:

- What are the primary environmental health concerns within Indian country and Alaska Native villages?

- What are the existing environmental health research needs within Indian country and Alaska Native villages?

- What is needed to provide for an effective environmental health program and research agenda within Indian country and Alaska Native villages?

- What role should the Environmental Protection Agency have in developing and supporting an environmental health program and research agenda within Indian country and Alaska Native villages?

- What agencies or organizations need to be involved in creating and implementing an effective environmental health research agenda within Indian country and Alaska Native villages?

Although the IPS was not able to formulate answers for all of these questions, the following observations and recommendations flow from the IPS' examination of these issues.

A. **INFRASTRUCTURE**

The health and environment of many AI/AN communities are adversely affected by critical infrastructure deficiencies involving essential functions such as the provision of safe drinking water, the safe treatment of wastewater and solid waste, and effective and equitable environmental regulation and enforcement. In simple terms, AI/ANs suffer a disproportionately high incidence of illness, injury, and disease directly attributable to the inadequacy or absence of proper facilities or environmental regulatory programs. These deficiencies flow principally from inadequate technical and financial assistance, including a continuing lack of such resources for designing, developing, and implementing environmental health research programs for Indian country and Alaska Native villages.

Although the Environmental Protection Agency leads federal efforts in protecting the environment within Indian country and Alaska Native villages, the Indian Health Service is the principal federal health care provider and health advocate for AI/ANs. The provision of these health-related services arise from the trust responsibility and special government-to-government relationship between the federal government and federally recognized Indian tribes. Currently, the Indian Health Service is funded and staffed at only 34% of the level of need. The IPS believes that this level of funding is shameful and utterly inadequate to meet the environmental and general health needs of Indian country and Alaska Native villages.

The fact that AI/AN communities persist as some of the most impoverished areas of the nation, coupled with the trust responsibility owed by the United States to federally recognized tribal governments, should compel the federal government to meet and fund essential environmental and health needs in Indian country and Alaska Native villages fully and immediately. Accordingly, with respect to infrastructure, the IPS recommends that the Administrator of the Environmental Protection Agency take the following actions:

1. Support legislative initiatives, including but not limited to the reauthorization of the Indian Health Care Improvement Act, that will eliminate inequities in federal funding to address the alarmingly high levels of unmet environmental and health needs of AI/ANs, regardless of where they live.

2. Promote the federal policy of tribal self-determination and self-sufficiency by building the environmental protection and environmental health capabilities of federally recognized tribes so that they can participate fully and effectively in the protection of the human health and environment of AI/AN communities.

3. Direct the Interagency Working Group on Environmental Justice, in collaboration with federally recognized tribes, to use its Roundtable on Environmental Justice in Indian Country as a model or vehicle for identifying possible strategies to address unmet environmental health and research needs in Indian country and Alaska Native villages promptly, effectively, and equitably.

4. Assert a leadership role among federal agencies in developing new financing mechanisms and leveraging all available resources to fund and implement environmental health-related projects and research in Indian country and Alaska Native villages.

5. Support innovative and sustainable technologies within Indian country and Alaska Native villages (*e.g.*, waterless toilets, solar energy systems, and constructed wetlands).

6. In collaboration with other federal agencies, ensure adequate priority funding and technical assistance for the design, construction, and operation of safe drinking water, sanitation, and wastewater facilities to protect all AI/AN communities whose health is imminently threatened by the absence or inadequacy of such facilities.

B. ENVIRONMENTAL HEALTH RESEARCH / DATA

Unfortunately, the overall status of environmental health within Indian country and Alaska Native villages is unknown. It also appears that there is no cohesive body of baseline data on environmental health issues affecting AI/AN communities, nor any ongoing, over-arching, collaborative effort by any entity to develop one. In a few areas such as solid waste disposal and cleanup, a federal, multi-agency workgroup is being used to help tribes bring their solid waste disposal sites into compliance with federal law. However, such collaborative efforts by federal agencies are the exception, not the rule. Moreover, in other critical areas, federal agency action to assess specific environmental health conditions in AI/AN communities, such as conducting a complete inventory of hazardous waste sites within Indian country and Alaska Native villages or determining contamination levels in subsistence foods, appears to be minimal if occurring at all.

Identifying the various environmental exposures affecting each AI/AN community should be an ongoing task, undertaken in consultation with federally recognized tribes. Specifically, data about the susceptibilities of AI/AN communities to various environmental agents is needed to help these communities understand and ameliorate some of their excess and disproportionate risk of exposure. In sum, a coordinated effort among federal, tribal, and state governments is needed to improve the collection and dissemination of environmental health information within Indian country and Alaska Native villages and to link it effectively with specific communities of concern. Toward that end, the IPS recommends that the Administrator of the Environmental Protection Agency take the following actions in collaboration with other appropriate federal agencies:

1. Support regional meetings and a national summit of federal agencies, federally recognized tribes, and concerned tribal organizations to discuss the environmental health needs of AI/AN and design a comprehensive environmental health research agenda to address those needs.

2. Consult with federally recognized tribes and involve members of AI/AN communities in designing, planning, and implementing specific environmental health research that reflects not only the traditional and cultural practices of such communities, but also their needs and concerns.

3. Ensure that environmental health research data is reported back to tribal governments and AI/AN communities promptly and in an understandable manner.

4. Preserve the confidentiality of the individuals who contribute to environmental health research data, protect such data from release under the Freedom of Information Act to the greatest extent permitted under federal law, and ensure that federally recognized tribal governments and AI/AN communities understand fully that some data may be made public.

5. Identify the benefit of the research to the tribal government before, during, and after the completion of the environmental health research.

6. Ensure that researchers obtain all approvals from the appropriate tribal government and/or its delegated review board before conducting any environmental health research.

7. Review available baseline environmental health data for Indian country and Native Alaska villages and take prompt steps to remedy all data insufficiencies.

8. Retain and store environmental and health data on each federally recognized tribal government and provide a means for each tribe to access easily the information applicable to its members and territory.

9. Request that the Indian Health Service make its annual data on health status readily available to each federally recognized tribe and other federal agencies.

10. In consultation with federally recognized tribes and with the involvement of concerned tribal organizations, conduct environmental research, studies, and monitoring programs to determine the effects on, and ways to mitigate the effects on the health of AI/AN communities due to exposure to environmental hazards, including but not limited to persistent organic pollutants and persistent bioaccumulative and toxic pollutants, nuclear resource development, uranium and other mine tailing deposits, petroleum contamination, and contamination of the water source and/or food chain. This is critical where the health of such communities is particularly susceptible to environmental harm because they are known to rely on subsistence hunting, fishing, and gathering.

11. Where appropriate, include state and local governments in collaborative efforts to collect environmental and health data relevant to Indian country and Alaska Native villages. For example, state environmental protection agencies may have access to monitoring information on off-reservation facilities that may be causing or contributing to adverse health consequences in AI/AN communities located nearby, down-stream, and/or down-wind.

C. COLLABORATION AND COORDINATION

Through its Policy for the Administration of Environmental Programs on Indian Reservations ("Indian Policy"), dated November 8, 1984, the Environmental Protection Agency vowed to give special consideration to tribal interests in making policy, to recognize tribal governments as the primary decision makers for environmental matters on reservations, to encourage cooperation between tribal, state, and local governments in resolving common environmental concerns, and to work with other federal agencies that have related responsibilities to help tribes assume environmental program responsibilities.

In several instances, there has been a reduction or even elimination of financial and technical resources from federal programs serving Indian country and Alaska Native villages. Accordingly, interagency collaboration and coordination are crucial for ensuring that limited federal financial and technical resources are used effectively and efficiently to address tribal environmental and health issues. This is increasingly important as tribes strive to build their own environmental and public health programs.

Some efforts at interagency collaboration have occurred. For example, in June 1991, the Bureau of Indian Affairs, the Environmental Protection Agency, the Department of Housing and Urban Development, and the Indian Health Service signed a Memorandum of Understanding ("MOU"), which recognizes that each agency has responsibilities and interests regarding the protection of human health and the environment as it relates to pollution control and prevention within Indian country and Alaska Native villages. This national MOU identifies areas of mutual interest, encourages coordination to promote the most effective and integrated use of the agencies' resources, and expressly anticipates that regional and area offices of the signatory agencies may want to develop more specific MOUs. Despite the MOU's laudable goals, the IPS has been unable to determine the full extent of its use and overall success or failure during the last nine years. However, the IPS has learned that tribal leaders and participating federal agencies at the 1999 EPA/Tribal Leaders' Summit in Denver, Colorado concluded that a regional MOU should be developed to address environmental protection issues within Indian country. In early 2000, a new regional MOU ("MOU 2000") was developed and executed by a broader group of federal agencies that work on tribal environmental issues within the Environmental Protection Agency's Region 8 geographic area. Signatories to the MOU 2000 hope that it will serve as "a demonstration initiative to develop and test new approaches to cooperation and coordination that may have national application."[22]

Presidential Executive Order 12898, "Federal Actions to Address Environmental Justice in Minority Populations and Low-Income Populations," dated February 11, 1994, calls upon all federal agencies to focus on the environmental and human health conditions in minority and low-income communities and in AI/AN communities. To coordinate the efforts of federal agencies to implement this directive, the Executive Order created an Interagency Working Group on Environmental Justice ("IWG"). During the last year, the IWG developed the "Integrated Federal Interagency Environmental Justice Action Agenda." The Agenda seeks to encourage greater collaboration and coordination among federal agencies to address environmental and public health concerns by demonstrating, through a set of projects, the benefits of having federal agencies collaborate to achieve environmental justice. The IWG conducted one of these projects, "Environmental Justice in Indian Country: A Roundtable to Address Conceptual, Political, and Statutory Issues," in Albuquerque, New Mexico on May 3-4, 2000. The Roundtable provided an opportunity for dialogue between federal agencies, tribal representatives, tribal organizations, and other interested parties on conceptual, political, and statutory issues of environmental justice in Indian country. A final report on the results of the Roundtable is expected to be available in Fall 2000. The IPS hopes that this effort will serve as a foundation for continuing efforts to build sustainable partnerships promoting health and environmental justice within Indian country and Alaska Native villages.

In sum, although the MOU and IWG are worthy efforts in principle, as a practical and general matter, the federal environmental and public health programs, projects, and activities now serving Indian country and Alaska Native villages are not coordinated effectively between the federal agencies. With this in mind, the IPS recommends that the Administrator of the Environmental Protection Agency take the following actions in collaboration with other appropriate federal agencies:

1. Because federal environmental missions and resources are divided among and in some cases overlap between various agencies, coordinate and pool available technical and financial resources to provide environmental health-related services to federally recognized tribes equitably, efficiently, and effectively. Towards this end, the Bureau of Indian Affairs, Environmental Protection Agency, Department of Housing and Urban Development, and the Indian Health Service should appraise the usefulness and implementation of the national MOU, *previously discussed*, and take appropriate steps to enhance and better promote interagency coordination and collaboration pertaining to the protection of health and the environment within Indian country and Alaska Native villages. The MOU 2000 may serve as a model for better implementing these efforts at regional and local Indian country and Alaska Native village levels. Additionally,

interested tribes should be considered appropriate parties to similar regional MOUs addressing the protection of health and the environment on their particular reservations.

2. Make regulatory decisions and develop federal policies affecting the health of AI/AN communities in consultation with federally recognized tribes. To the greatest extent possible, such decisions should be based not only science, but also should address and incorporate the traditional knowledge of the AI/AN community. For example, limitations on the consumption of traditional foods due to pollution danger may trigger unique social, economic, and health problems within AI/AN communities.

3. Be proactive in helping federally recognized tribes identify financial and technical resources throughout the federal government to address their environmental concerns and related health needs. By marshaling all available resources, federal agencies can promote "one-stop" shopping for tribal environmental and health-related programs and transcend traditional agency boundaries.

4. Use all available means to increase access by federally recognized tribes and AI/AN communities to federal environmental and health-related programs, services, financial and technical resources, and data bases, including but not limited to the use of publications, training and technical assistance, and Internet postings.

5. In consultation with federally recognized tribes, develop a federally-funded, comprehensive, interagency program on environmental health that will address fully the environmental justice needs within Indian country and Alaska Native villages.

6. Expand current agency definitions of "environmental health" to incorporate an active federal health role in tribal environmental programs, including pollution prevention, mitigation, and remediation within Indian country and Alaska Native villages. This recommendation is particularly relevant to the Indian Health Service's current view of "environmental health."

7. Whenever possible and appropriate, include state and local governments in collaborative efforts to address human health and environmental justice issues within Indian country and Alaska Native villages. Because pollution does not respect jurisdictional boundaries, collaborative efforts in the human health and environmental justice arena similarly should eclipse political differences. Additionally, states must be swayed to incorporate environmental justice principles and goals into their laws, policies, and practices.

8. Encourage states to increase and promote access by federally recognized tribes and AI/AN communities to all available state environmental and health-related programs, services, resources, and data bases, including but not limited to creating a resource inventory of state benefits that are available to tribes and AI/AN communities. For example, a state should be strongly encouraged to make available to tribes and AI/ANs

those state financial and technical resources and services otherwise available to non-Native citizens and communities within that state.

D. TRAINING AND EDUCATION

To fulfill the federal government's trust responsibility owed to federally recognized tribes and to understand the protocol for working with tribes on a government-to-government basis in all matters that may affect tribal interests, it is critical that federal agency staff and managers be trained in federal Indian law, the history of federal Indian policies and legislation, and tribal culture and government. Although the Environmental Protection Agency has made significant strides through its "Working Effectively with Tribal Governments" training course, the training of staff and managers has been inconsistent throughout the agency. For example, while some program offices have trained a majority of their staff for work with tribal governments, other offices have made only cursory efforts. Training and education on environmental justice and environmental hazards within Indian country and Alaska Native villages also is needed at the federal and tribal governmental levels and within AI/AN communities. Finally, in most cases, state governments also should be included in these efforts to promote a better understanding by state officials of these issues and principles.

Based on the foregoing considerations, the IPS recommends that the Administrator of the Environmental Protection Agency take the following actions concerning training and education in collaboration with other appropriate federal agencies:

1. Ensure that agency staff and managers have a thorough understanding of federal Indian law and policies, tribal culture, and the unique governmental structure of federally recognized Indian tribes, including Alaska Native villages. This is particularly important for those people directly working on these issues.

2. Incorporate training into each environmental health research project so that, upon completion, trained personnel will remain in the AI/AN community to promote and monitor the environmental health of the community members on a long term and continuing basis.

3. Focus education efforts on environmental justice and the cause, effect, and remediation of specific environmental hazards. These efforts also should strive to improve the understanding of these issues among AI/AN communities and health professionals serving these communities, including but not limited to medical, nursing, and public health practitioners.

4. Increase the number of professionals specializing in environmental health issues confronting AI/AN communities. Because persons who have been exposed to certain hazardous substances such as lead, mercury, pesticides, TCE, and PCBs are at risk for developing permanent disabilities or diseases such as intelligence and behavioral impairments, endocrine disruptions, and cancer, the Indian Health Service, in particular, should be strongly encouraged to focus on preventing these exposures among AI/ANs,

monitoring and educating AI/ANs whose health is at risk due to pollution and hazardous substance exposure, and providing equitable and fair medical treatment and long-term assistance to affected AIANs.

5. Assist tribes in developing tools, processes, and technical resources to assess better the overall justness of economic development projects proposed for their lands, including but not limited to identifying potential impacts on human health and the environment and on pollution prevention initiatives.

1. See Executive Memorandum on Government-to-Government Relations with Native American Tribal Governments (April 29, 1994).

2. See Executive Order No. 13084 (May 14, 1998).

3. "Federally recognized" means that these tribes and groups have a special legal relationship with the United States. Additionally, a number of tribes and indigenous groups do not have federally recognized status, although some of these tribes are state-recognized or are in the process of seeking federal recognition.

4. AI/ANs are among the fastest growing ethnic/minority populations in the nation. The 1990 census showed a 37.9% increase over the population of AI/ANs in the 1980 census. For additional facts and general information, see the Bureau of Indian Affairs' homepage at <http://www.doi.gov/bia/aitoday/q_and_a.html>.

5. For additional facts and general information, see the Bureau of Indian Affairs' homepage at <http://www.doi.gov/bia/aitoday/q_and_a.html>.

6. The term "Indian country" is defined by federal law as including "(a) all land within the limits of any Indian reservation under the jurisdiction of the United States Government, notwithstanding the issuance of any patent, and, including rights of way running through the reservation, (b) all dependent Indian communities . . . and (c) all Indian allotments, the Indian titles to which have not been extinguished, including rights-of-way running through the same." See 18 U.S.C. § 1151.

7. See, e.g., "National Gambling Impact Study Commission Report, Chapter 6, titled *Native American Tribal Gambling*, at page 6-5 (June 18, 1999).

8. Id.

9. See, e.g., The Forgotten America -- Alaska's Rural Sanitation Problem, a Video Produced by The Media Support Center for the Alaska Department of Environmental Conservation.

10. Id.

11. See, e.g., Wallwork Winik, Lyric, "There's A New Generation with a Different Attitude," Parade Magazine at 6-7 (July 18, 1999).

12. Proposed IHCA Amendments of 2000, Section 2(h), prepared by the National Steering Committee for the Reauthorization of the Indian Health Care Improvement Act, P.L. 94-437 (October 6, 1999), and based on data used by the Indian Health Service for the FY 2001 budget development.

13. See National Cancer Institute, National Institute of Health, HHS, Office of Special Populations Research Web Site, "The Cancer Burden," at <http://ospr.nci.nih.gov.burden.htm>.

14. K. Marie Porterfield, "American Indian Cancer Statistics Under Reported," Indian Country Today at C-1 (July 26, 2000).

15. See "Focus on American Indian and Alaska Native Populations," published by the Agency for Toxic Substances and Disease Registry, at pages 1-2.

16. For example, tribes near the Hanford Nuclear Reservation have been working with the Agency for Toxic Substances and Disease Registry to design health assessments focusing on exposure effects from food consumption and other activities. These tribes want to learn if the Hanford releases affect native food items and local materials used in tribal products like storage and cooking baskets, mats, and clothing. See "Focus on American Indian and Alaska Native Populations," published by the Agency for Toxic Substances and Disease Registry, at page 5. Tribes located in coastal northern California are concerned about the pesticide exposure of some 300 traditional basketmakers who gather their own materials from the forests and roadsides. Because a disproportionate number of American Indian residents in Humboldt County, California have been diagnosed with cancer, tribes believe studies are needed to determine the exact cause of such cases. See Chuck Striplen, Mutzun Oholone Tribe, "Native Subsistence in a Toxic Environment: A Tribal Viewpoint," at page 14, EPA's OPPTS Tribal News (Fall/Winter 1999-2000).

17. A number of studies have shown that children are uniquely susceptible to pollution and contaminants. For example, since 1992, the Agency for Toxic Substances and Disease Registry has funded research in the Great Lakes states focusing on the health effects of high risk populations, including American Indians, from persistent toxic substances found in fish. One study found that newborns born to mothers who consumed only 2.3 PCB-contaminated Great Lakes fish meals per month scored lower on the Neonatal Behavioral Assessment Scale. See "Focus on American Indian and Alaska Native Populations," published by the Agency for Toxic Substances and Disease Registry, at pages 2-3. Additionally, in Oklahoma, Indian children also suffer harm from their environment. The Tar Creek Superfund Site, a former lead and zinc mine, occupies 40 square miles within the boundaries of the former Quapaw Indian Reservation. Both the Quapaw Tribe's powwow grounds and campgrounds are contaminated from mine tailings, and the Environmental Protection Agency Region 6 reports that approximately 25% of the Quapaw children have elevated blood lead levels compared with a statewide average of 2%. See "U.S. Environmental Protection Agency Region 6 Environmental Justice Update," at page 7 (May 2000).

18. See, e.g., City of Albuquerque v. Browner, 97 F.3d 415 (10th Cir. 1996), cert. denied, 118 S. Ct. 410 (1997) (upholding the Environmental Protection Agency's approval of the Pueblo of Isleta's water quality standards that were more stringent than the state water quality standards, and which included a ceremonial use standard).

19. Since 1986, the Safe Drinking Water Act, Clean Water Act, and Clean Air Act have been amended to afford tribes substantially the same opportunities as states to assume

responsibility for certain programs or purposes.

20.   For example, the Environmental Protection Agency recently reported that, as of July 13, 2000, only 15 tribes have Environmental Protection Agency-approved or -promulgated water quality standards and no tribes are authorized to administer the National Pollutant Discharge Elimination System or to establish Total Maximum Daily Loads. <u>See</u> 65 Fed. Reg. 43,585 (July 13, 2000).

21.   For example, a New York State Department of Health study of lactating women and their infants linked breast feeding and infant exposure to hazardous substances. This study compared PCB levels in the breast milk of Mohawk women who gave birth between 1986 and 1992 with a control group. The study found that although the PCB concentrations in the breast milk of Mohawk mothers decreased over time, their infants had urine PCB levels ten times higher than that of their mothers. <u>See</u> "Focus on American Indian and Alaska Native Populations," published by the Agency for Toxic Substances and Disease Registry, at pages 3-4. <u>See also</u> Winona Laduke, <u>All Our Relations, Native Struggles for Land and Life</u>, at 11-23 (1999).

22.   <u>See</u> MOU 2000 at Section I.